CRISIS INTERVENTION

TOPICAL SERIES IN COMMUNITY -CLINICAL PSYCHOLOGY

Series Editors

William L. Claiborn
Department of Psychology
University of Maryland
College Park

Robert Cohen
Institute for Community Development
110 Harvard Place
Syracuse, New York

William L. Claiborn & Robert Cohen
SCHOOL INTERVENTION

Gerald Specter & William L. Claiborn
CRISIS INTERVENTION

IN PREPARATION:

Robert Cohen & William L. Claiborn
WORKING WITH POLICE AGENCIES

Dorothy A. Evans & William L. Claiborn
MENTAL HEALTH SERVICES FOR THE POOR

CRISIS INTERVENTION
VOLUME TWO
A Topical Series in Community-Clinical Psychology

Edited by
Gerald A. Specter Ph.D. & William L. Claiborn Ph.D.
Department of Psychology
University of Maryland
College Park

Behavioral Publications   **New York**

Library of Congress Catalog Number 73-4360
ISBN:0-87705-118-6—clothbound
    0-87705-124-0—paperback
Copyright 1973 by Behavioral Publications

BEHAVIORAL PUBLICATIONS, Inc.
72 Fifth Ave.
New York, New York 10011

Printed in the United States of America

Second Printing

LIBRARY OF CONGRESS CATALOGING IN PUBLICATION DATA

Crisis intervention.

    (Topical series in community-clinical psychology [2])
    Papers presented at a symposium sponsored by the
University of Maryland, Mar. 23-25, 1972.
    1. Community mental health services—Congresses.
2. Psychotherapy—Congresses. I. Specter, Gerald A., ed.
II. Claiborn, William L., ed. III. Maryland. University.
IV. Series.
[DNLM: 1. Crisis intervention—Congresses. WM 420
C932 1972]
RA790.A1C77   362.2'2   73-4360

Contributing Authors

Philip Berck
Department of Psychology
University of California
Los Angeles, California

Alan L. Berman, Ph.D.
Assistant Professor of Psychiatry
Counselor, Counseling Center
American University
Washington, D.C.

Gail Bleach, M.A.
Department of Psychology
University of Maryland
College Park, Maryland

Elaine A. Blechman, Ph.D.
Department of Psychology
University of Maryland
College Park, Maryland

Gilbert Freitag, Ph.D.
Department of Psychology
University of California
Los Angeles, California

John Giddings, Ph.D.
Pittsburgh Child Guidance Center
Pittsburgh, Pennsylvania

Sondra Goldstein, Ph.D.
Pittsburgh Child Guidance Center
Pittsburgh, Pennsylvania

Dennis T. Jaffe
Number Nine 266 State St.
New Haven, Connecticut

Ija N. Korner, Ph.D.
University of Wisconsin at Green Bay
Green Bay, Wisconsin

Leo Levy, Ph.D., S.M. Hygiene
Department of Preventive Medicine &
    Community Health
University of Illinois at the
    Medical Center
Chicago, Illinois

Ann S. McColskey, Ph.D.
Clinical Psychologist
Pensacola, Florida

Nancy Sebolt, A.C.S.W.
Western Missouri Mental Health Center
Kansas City, Missouri

Edwin S. Shneidman, Ph.D.
Professor of Medical Psychology
Department of Psychiatry
University of California at Los Angeles
Los Angeles, California

Sam Stern, M.A.
Tuscaloosa Community Crisis Center
    and Department of Psychology
University of Alabama
Tuscaloosa, Alabama

Jon Williams, Ph.D.
Private Practice
9006 Eastbourne Lane
Laurel, Maryland 20810

Contents

This book is the second in a series of collections of papers from symposia on current issues in community-clinical psychology. In each volume an attempt has been made to select a
sampling of papers representing historical perspectives, current
practice, innovative programs, theoretical and conceptual ad-
vances and guidelines for training and evaluation.

The second annual symposium in Community-Clinical psychology,
supported by the University of Maryland, was held in College
Park, March 23-25, 1972. Participants totaled 126 from far
states and nearby communities. The symposium format included
presentation of formal papers, discussions, participatory work-
shops and informal sessions. The formal papers appear in this
volume intact. Dr. Shneidman opened the conference with informal remarks which set the tone for the sessions, and later
presented a videotape and discussion on "the crisis of death".
His opening remarks are presented in Chapter 1. Dr. Berman
translated his experiential workshop into a helpful chapter on
training of hotline workers. Dennis Jaffe led an extended discussion on "the case of Sara" which can be found in a more formal version in his chapter. The contributions of Al Engelman and
Berkley Hathorne did not permit presentation in written form.
The former was an active participatory study of organizational
and social crises and the latter was an. enlightening discussion
of a film on a suicide used for training of suicidologists.

Hopefully much of the learning from the symposium came from
the interaction of the participants with the more formal structure. These personal learnings can not be reflected directly in
the volume, but hopefully readers will find much to stimulate
their conceptualization and practice, and to enhance the quality
of debate and discussion on the issues. The book reflects a
symposium organized around crisis intervention strategies; it is
seen as appropriate for current practitioners, administrators,
"participant-conceptualizers," researchers, and students.

Like all such endeavors, the final production of this volume
has depended upon the contributions of many individuals. The
symposium could not have been held without the support of C. J.
Bartlett, Ph.D., Chairman, Department of Psychology and F. B.

Tyler, Ph.D. Director of The Clinical Training Program, Department of Psychology, University of Maryland, College Park. The contributions of the participants, contributing authors, volume editors, and Mrs. Irma Nicholson were equally essential.

William L. Claiborn
Robert Cohen
Series Editors
College Park
December, 1972

I: INTRODUCTION

Crisis intervention might variously be described as a theoretical model, a clinical technique or even a social movement. As a theoretical model, crisis intervention still rests heavily upon the early formulations of Lindemann (1944) and subsequent elaborations by Caplan (1964). As a clinical technique, crisis intervention represents a strategy often employed, or at least advocated, but rarely assessed and refined. Viewed as a social movement, crisis intervention seems to be one expression of the general cultural trend toward seeking novel solutions to the problems of personal isolation in a fast-moving and often indifferent society. This book contains the proceedings of a symposium conducted at the University of Maryland which brought people together whose primary conceptions of crisis intervention spanned the range of possibilities. The symposium participants included academicians, who often showed a high degree of interest in theoretical issues, mental health program administrators, who frequently had particular concerns regarding implementation techniques, and, finally, front-line crisis workers who were often most involved with the personal and humanistic implications of crisis intervention. In some measure, it was the goal of the conference to bring together these people with their varying perspectives so that they might gain from a process of sharing.

At the close of the symposium on which this book is based, a participant was heard to comment that the conference might well have been a historical "last." He expressed the conviction that crisis work had entered the operational stage in which "doers" no longer would be greatly concerned with the output of thinkers and researchers. Viewing crisis intervention as a social phenomenon, the attractiveness of this conclusion is difficult to deny. The rapid proliferation of crisis centers, telephone hotlines and the like has not been paralleled by the emergence of a substantial literature on the theory and assessment of interventive programs. Moreover mistrust and

1

antagonism between academicians, full-time clinicians and paraprofessional workers is a real phenomenon which cannot be dis-
regarded. Even so, it remains to be hoped that crisis intervention need not become the domain of a particular group to the
exclusion of others with different perspectives. There are
some hopeful signs that the field may yet see reunion of fac-
tions which will result in better conceptualized, better imple-
mented and more humanly useful programs of service.

One obstacle to the full integration of the mental health
professional into the crisis intervention movement stems from
the theoretical bias which has dominated the professions. The
disease model under which professionals have generally been
trained tends to view breakdowns in psychological functioning
as manifestations of an underlying disease (Szasz, 1960). The
implication of this model is that psychological distress requires specialized treatment aimed at curing the illness by some-
how altering the defective personality. In contrast, crisis
theory as articulated by Lindemann (1944) and Caplan (1964)
assumes that an individual's resistance to stress is finite and
idiosyncratic, so that any person will, under certain circumstances, find his coping mechanisms inadequate to sustain his
psychological equilibrium. The treatment approach suggested
by this latter model would involve efforts to supplement the
personal resources of the individual who is failing under stress,
as opposed to efforts to ferret out a disease process. The
notion of supplementing resources in times of crisis also im-
plies that the interventionist need not possess specialized
techniques, but may usefully offer the human qualities of
warmth and empathy which ordinarily enable one person to provide support for another. This implication, in turn, may threaten the status needs of the professional who would prefer to
view himself as the possessor of a special magic for the alleviation of human suffering.

The development of the field of crisis intervention, thus,
comes to rest partially upon a fundamentally difficult choice
for the professional. Acceptance of the crisis model may require the partial or complete abandonment of some of the funda-
mental assumptions in which he is trained and, further, may require him to develop new and less exclusive skills for intervention. Yet if the mental health professional declines to
alter his views and actions, he may be left behind by enthusias-
tic non-professionals who see a chance to be humanly useful,
with or without the help of highly trained personnel. It is
encouraging to note that most of the contributors to the book
are professionally trained individuals who have, in varying de-
grees, committed themselves to the crisis intervention model.

This last point, encouraging though it may be with relation

to the entry of professionals into the field, might also be
viewed as disturbing with regard to the emerging role of the
non-professional. Only one paper included in the collection
(that of Mr. Jaffe) was written by an individual who neither
possessed nor was seeking an advanced degree in one of the
mental health professions. This fact may be partially reflective of the academic biases which affected paper selection.
It may also be the case, however, that service oriented non-
professional workers have less commitment to the evaluation and
communication of their experiences, less ability to organize
and convey their thinking, and/or less access to the media of
communication. Insofar as any or all of these hypotheses are
valid, the non-professional worker may still have great need
of the professional if he wishes to facilitate the emergence
and evolution of new programs.

The foregoing discussion of the uncertainties and difficulties which currently challenge the crisis intervention movement
leads inevitably to a question: Is the new model a passing fad
which will die out when the enthusiasm of its innovators dimin-
ishes? Will crisis intervention join moral therapy, insulin
shock therapy and psychosurgery as an approach which had its
day and then largely disappeared? The danger of this is real
enough, whether or not the treatment model is valid; 19th cent-
ury moral therapy, for example, died out as a treatment mode
not because it was shown to be ineffectual, but because it was
supplanted by better articulated and more "scientific" types
of therapy reflecting the changing Zeitgeist (Zax and Specter,
In press). The same fate may befall the crisis approach, with
the possibility that new techniques will supplant it, or that
traditional methods and concepts will prevail.

A crucial issue in considering whether the crisis model
will persist or prevail concerns the degree to which programs
of crisis intervention may achieve institutionalized stability.
Small, poorly funded and largely unreported programs are unlikely to sustain a major movement. On the other hand, programs
which become integral parts of substantial mental health facilities may gain the crisis intervention approach vital public
recognition and financial support. Some impetus for institutionalized crisis services was provided by the well-known report of the Joint Commission on Mental Illness and Health (1961).
That report, based upon a massive analysis of the nation's mental health care establishment, recommended the creation of
multi-service community-based facilities. Among the types of
service which the Commission strongly endorsed was the provision
of immediate emergency care. The Commission advocated the rapid
expansion and extension of such services in existing facilities
as well as in new centers. Scrutiny of the Report does not

suggest that the Commission members were advocating the crisis
model as such. Indeed, the wording of the document, which
includes references to the "acutely ill" leaves no doubt that
the proposal was thoroughly consistent with the traditional
disease model. Nevertheless, the operationalized efforts to
provide emergency care inevitably opened the doors of the mental health center to a wide range of individuals in crisis. It
is a practical impossibility to provide well publicized, accessible facilities and then bar from entry people whose crisis responses do not fit the established categories of illness. Thus,
many community mental health centers have come to incorporate
crisis services structurally similar to those outside of the institutional milieu. The question remains, however, as to
whether such institutional crisis services will generally evolve
toward the newer conceptual framework, or will ultimately become mere admissions screening units to inpatient services where
traditional therapies are utilized.

Another issue relevant to the lasting power of the crisis
intervention movement concerns the willingness of funding agencies to support innovative efforts. In this regard, the authors
are less optimistic. As judged, for example, by research grants
issued by the National Institutes of Health crisis intervention
is no longer the "hot" field that it was as recently as two or
three years ago. There is as yet no evidence that numerous
existing programs are failing due to lack of funds, but the financial climate would not seem to favor the emergence of new
projects.

A final consideration relevant to the future of crisis intervention provides a more promising picture. Grass roots support for the approach may well be extensively generated by the
large numbers of people who have the opportunity to·serve as
front-line crisis workers. Even a poorly funded telephone hotline on a small college campus may operate with a large volunteer staff. To the extent that crisis work is productive and
satisfying, these centers may send forth armies of people who
understand and favor the approach. In particular, the college
crisis facilities may provide an attractive experience for
students seeking careers in the mental health professions, thus
generating a later sample of professionals already familiar with
the model. More traditional therapeutic approaches are less
likely to gain adherents through this process, because the skill
level required obviates the possibility that large numbers of
undergraduates could personally sample the job role of the therapist. (The impact of this last point must be tempered, however by the observation that considering the extremely high
numbers of students seeking admission to post graduate mental
health training, careers involving traditional therapies remain

relatively attractive to college students even in the absence of opportunities to serve as therapists.)

The balance of this book may be viewed as providing a sample of the issues and efforts in crisis intervention. The uninitiated reader must conclude for himself whether the promises and challenges of the crisis model, as illustrated, warrant the support or abandonment of the approach. It is the editors' belief that the ultimate success of most projects in community psychology depends upon the ability of the innovator to explain and justify his efforts. Regardless of internal difficulties and conceptual debates, support of crisis intervention services will rise or fall on the tides of public sentiments. Hopefully, the contents of this book will broaden the professional, strengthen the novice, and stimulate the administrator.

The chapters reflect the evolution of theory, the state of the clinical art, guidelines for organization, suggestions for training, ideas for technique, and advocacy of empirical research. In the long run when the fad fades, public support will be sustained only by proven success. These authors' contributions can be utilized by many diversely functioning crisis intervenors to build and evaluate quality theory and practice.

Crisis intervention represents a new opportunity filled with uncertainties and badly mounted efforts. Yet the promise remains, and it might well be society's loss if the potentials remain unexplored due to the failure of the crisis interventionists to make their case heard.

REFERENCES

Caplan, G. *Principles of preventive psychiatry*. New York: Basic Books, 1964.

Joint Commission on Mental Illness and Health. *Action for mental health*. New York: Science Editions, 1961.

Lindemann, E. Symptomatology and management of acute grief. *American Journal of Psychiatry*, 1944, *101*, 141-148.

Szasz, T. S. The myth of mental illness. *American Psychologist*, 1960, *15*, 113-118.

Zax, M. & Specter, G. *Community Psychology: A Text*. New York: Wiley, In press.

II: CONCEPTS

Edwin Shneidman is perhaps the best known of the Suicidologists and is a logical choice for opening remarks about crisis intervention strategies. While Caplan and Lindemann are credited with major impact in the field, Shneidman has been closely involved with the operationalization of a major direct attack on one clear crisis: suicide. His general model of crisis prevades most modern attempts at management of immediate crisis.

Theory has had too little influence on practice in crisis intervention: models seem nearly unable to keep up with newly evolving techniques which exist and survive, at least momentarily, because of their psychological attractiveness. As yet, we have no broad yet specific unifying theory of crisis that is both testable and a generator of intervention strategies. In this section the chapters by Korner and Levy deal with some aspects of the theory problem though they focus more intensely on the personal aspects of each authors' work. The three chapters do, however, provide examples of the way in which participant conceptualizers use theory to generate practice, and practice to stimulate theory.

1: PERSPECTIVES

Dr. Shneidman has written extensively and intensively on crisis intervention. Much of what appears in this chapter can be found with considerable elaboration elsewhere. However, these remarks, edited from the opening talk of the conference, provide a historical and philosophical outline for the reading and reviewing of the remaining chapters. Some of the concepts and principles which have painfully evolved through the Sturm and Drang of the recent decades are summarized.

The conceptualization of inter, intra and extra temporal crises helps a worker anticipate the development of predictable crises, and to generate crisis specific interventive strategies. Shneidman gently prods us to shake loose from our "professional" bias for arm chair theorizing in the face of a client's immediate intense crisis. (See also the chapter by Korner.) Many professionals need to be reminded that short term dependency (or transference) is not anathema, - but a human, natural response to stress. We often seem to confuse the individual's long run need for personal interdependence by labeling as pathological the appearance of initial strong dependency in a client in crisis.

Dr. Shneidman reminds the crisis worker of the dangers and the limitations inherent in a logical positivist outlook. Such a world view makes it difficult to respond effectively to the intense ambivalence evidenced by a person in crisis. For those of us who depend upon it for order and the control of anxiety in our own lives, it is a hard lesson.

Finally, Dr. Shneidman applauds the "democratization" of mental health crisis services, and notes the potential benefits of a society fostering democratic interdependence. We applaud this too, and the reader will note several instances in the following chapters in which the consequence of the intervention program is broader, less hierarchical and a less formal "service" to our fellow man in crisis.

CRISIS INTERVENTION: SOME THOUGHTS AND PERSPECTIVES

Edwin Shneidman

University of California at Los Angeles

There is a pleasantly grandiose aura that surrounds intensive, long-term psychotherapy. In that process, the magician, priest, physician, medicine man, psychologist, seer, healer, psychiatrist, therapist attempt to exorcise the devils, to cure the insanities, to reorganize and reconstitute the personality and to unblemish character. He aims at outcomes of heroic proportions. But, clearly, there is room for benign interventive processes with *less* extensive goals. Brief psychotherapy and crisis intervention are the major occupants of that obvious *terra incognito*.

Crisis intervention practice can be operationally defined in terms of the specific goal of restoring an individual to his pretraumatic level of overt functioning. Obviously, the occurrence of some external traumatic event is implied.

Crises can be usefully discussed in terms of two major dimensions: the time of life at which they occur, and the intensity or cataclysmic dimension of the event. Curiously, what is left out is the personality of the victim. Crisis intervention theories, in large part, are treatments of persons without a science of personology.

The torments of people in crisis are best conceptualized not as diseases and not as psychological disorders, but as sociopsychological blights or disasters. We need to look to new models -- essentially neo-Freudian ones. Following in the paths of Freud are the large steps of people like Kris, Hartman, Erikson and Holt. Each of these men working from the main corpus of psychoanalytic theory, has developed concepts relating especially to ego-functioning, and to the functioning of normal people in fairly normal situations. Erich Lindemann, in his all-important follow-up of the tragic (Boston) Coconut Grove fire, recognized that there could be other goals than that of reconstituting the character and the personality. Because of the pressure

of time and number, he addressed himself to the "survivor vic-
tims" of that fire. He called his helpful process "preventive
intervention," which I have labelled "postvention" (in that it
comes *after* the dire event). Lindemann recognized that there
were people who were in a state of psychological impotence,
numbness and shock and that his most important immediate function was to bring them back to where they were before the trauma,
to put them on their feet again, so to speak, and let them be
as they were before.

Over the past several years, Gerald Caplan, like Lindemann
at Harvard, and his students have contributed to the development
of crisis practice and theory. For example, Phyllis Rolfe Silverman has recently worked on widow-to-widow programs; "seasoned" survivor-victims helping fresh survivor-victims.

There are a number of systemic implications to this approach. One implication relates to the theory of causality. If
one thinks of a person, for example, who stutters, there is an
implied heirarchy of causes that goes something like this: precipitating causes, resonating and sustaining causes, reinforcing causes, and primary causes. The therapist would make it
his task to go to a "little lower layer," to use a Melvillian
phrase, and to uncover "deeper," perhaps the deepest, layers of
personality (dys) functioning. "Let's get at the roots," is a
way of saying, lets get at underlying, if not primary, causes.

Not so in crisis intervention. The crisis intervener is
content (because his goals are different) to deal primarily with
precipitating causes. If someone is shaking with anxiety after
an earthquake, one deals with the precipitant of the anxiety and
is content to mollify or reduce the intensity of that symptom
which resulted from that event. A natural disaster, an accident,
a traumatic death of a loved one, or some other event of great
magnitude, is obviously a situation that creates great psychological havoc. One can legitimately respond in terms of crisis
intervention. An event that comes quickly to mind is the atomic
bomb explosion at Hiroshima. (The book to read on that topic is
Robert Lifton's *Death in Life*).

If one listens to what happens in crisis intervention, one
hears a great deal more about the top layer of causes. As a
suicidologist, I am not deeply impressed when someone tells me
that the "causes" of suicide are divorce, being jilted, ill
health, having cancer, fearing cancer, loss of job, and so on.
Those are only the precipitating causes at best, and while those
are dire things to happen in a life, it is also true that the
vast majority of people who undergo those dire events do not
commit suicide. One cannot fully explain self-destructive phenomenon simply with talk about loss of a loved one, losing money,

and so on. But -- if you are going to practice crisis intervention, you can do just that. You can talk meaningfully about
those precipitants because it is precisely the effects of those
precipitants that you wish to undo. You need not aspire to do
more. That is one major characteristic of crisis theory.

A second major implication, which flows from that first one,
is that one does not necessarily need the same intensity of training that is required to do regular psychotherapy. What you need
is a good heart, freedom from proselytizing for your own private
causes, supervised training focused on crisis intervention and a
pinch of wisdom. Many people can usefully participate in a large
variety of crisis intervention activities. They can be non-professional volunteers. It is not just an accident that, in the
past decade, suicide prevention and crisis intervention centers
made use of volunteers; theoretically it was a hand-in-glove
situation. One cannot take a well-meaning woman in her thirties
or forties whose children are in school, whose husband is support-
ing his family, who is a mature person in her community, and expect to train her to do depth psychotherapy. There is too much
of a background of concepts, practices and facts to be mastered
to expect anyone to do that. But one can work with such a person
and within six months have an absolutely first-rate crisis intervener. Three pre-conditions are essential: *careful* selection;
rigorous training; and *continuous* ruthless, supervision.

A few general remarks: It has become part of our common
psychological lore to know about Erik Erikson's eight psycho-
sexual stages of development. Most of us are familiar with these
hypothesized stages in the development of the human psyche, and
with those conflicts we must resolve in order to go on to the
next step of our own psychological development. An even better
summary of the process is contained in Jacque's speech in *As You
Like it*. But we seem to age in spurts. Our lives, as far as our
feelings about our own "age", seem to move in this disjointed
way. When do you cease being an adolescent and become an adult?
When do you turn into middle age? When does old age start? The
questions are rhetorical. We move in spurts -- but there are
discernible differences in these different stages of life.

All this is background to saying that three kinds of crisis
can be distinguished. Some crises occur *during* a stage of life.
They are crises within adolescence, middle age, or old age. These
are called *intratemporal* crises. They are crises typical of that
time of life. In Goethe's *Sorrow of a Young Werther* one can see
what an adolescent crisis is about.

Oftentimes, a person can make it when he's doing what he's
been doing, but when it comes time for him to be pushed to the
next major task in his life, he has difficulty at the *turn* in

life. Many people can be adolescents quite successfully, but they have difficulty *becoming* adults. (It's as though you're in your car, driving down the highway on a Sunday afternoon, and there's the little woman with all the kids, one of whom has to go to the toilet, another has just dropped his ice cream cone down the back of your neck, someone is pointing to some scenery and happens to put his finger in your eye, etc. You can handle it all while you're on the straightaway, but if this happens when you're in a turn, you may be in trouble and go off the road). At a turn in life, the resistance to taking a new task can lead to *intertemporal* crises; crises that occur in the interstices between the major times of life. It's hard to become an old person; it's hard to become a middle aged person; it's hard to become a young adult; it's hard to become an adolescent and give up childhood. Always involved is the "giving up" and the adjustment to the new, the uncomfortable, the unknown.

The third type of crisis is *extratemporal*. It occurs rather independent of time of life. These extratemporal crises can account for the phenomenon of apparently unaccountable suicides–the cases where one wonders why he did it. The causes, even the precipitating causes, are difficult or impossible to discern -- almost as though there were no specific precipitant. Perhaps the cause is an extratemporal crisis, a kind of metacrisis or resonating crisis. Ordinary stage-fright can serve as an example: One is standing here, and one needs to step back from oneself and recognize that he is in trouble and cannot get out of the trouble by trying to push through his wall of anxiety. One cannot push through the anxiety and recover the lost (blocked) memory until he decreases the anxiety itself -- by relaxing, candidly admitting the anxiety, pausing to collect one's wits, or whatever.

When you see someone in a *metacritical* suicidal situation (represented by the phrase "free-floating feelings"), the therapeutic maneuver of choice is not to talk about the money or getting her back, or improving one's health, the task then is primarily one of rolling back the intensity of the general anxiety. Many crises appear to have no precipitant. The therapist needs to be concerned about anxiety itself.

There are some instructive psychological similarities between suicide prevention and crisis intervention. The first is that they are short-lived; their duration is relatively brief. Unless there is intervention, a *highly* lethal person will either be dead or the intensity of the crisis itself will fall away, or some other things will happen. Intense suicidality can last only for a relatively brief period of time before either bullet or affect is discharged. Suicidal crises -- and crises in general -- are of relatively brief duration.

In general, crisis theory has held that an "adequate" period of crisis intervention need not exceed three months or so. But this rule of thumb probably needs to be modified where a death is involved.

The crisis after the death of a loved one seems to last about a year, a special year in which the survivor is at special risk.   London psychiatrist, C. M. Parkes has compared widows of various ages with matched non-widowed cohorts and has found that the morbidity and mortality rates of widows are several times greater in that first year.   They are much more apt to get themselves killed in traffic, to die of pneumonia, to drink and not eat, to have an infarction, to commit suicide, to die of neglect, or to suffer a sudden- unexpected death, etc. Also, they are much more apt to be in the hospital requiring surgery for a variety of reasons.   That first year is dangerous -- psychodynamically laden.

A second characteristic of crises (suicidal crises included) is that they are usually dyadic.   A dyadic relationship is, of course, a two-person relationship: spouses, lovers, parent and child.   It follows that crisis intervention will not work as well as it might unless it involves the "significant other," -- the other half of the dyad.   This is different from the usual practice of psychotherapy. In crisis intervention, if you are going to help him, you may have to meet her; and sometimes see both together.   It is pointless to mollify his anxiety and do your psychotherapeutic best and then send him out to her to be turned up again in short order. If she is "suicidogenic," if she "hides" the gun under his mattress -- which has happened -- then you need to know that.   On the other hand, this awful person he had described may turn out to be your best auxilliary therapist. One needs to assess that too. At the beginning, one has to understand that crisis intervention is, at the least, a dyadic interplay and that one has to involve the other significant person -- and agencies of the community, as well.

A third characteristic of suicidal crises, but not necessarily of crises attending to natural disasters, is ambivalence. Through our language and habitual patterns of thought, we are thoroughly ingrained in the Aristotelian way of thinking. We have notions of what is logical and what is illogical. An object or event either is or it isn't. But the psychological life is not necessarily dichotomous. It typically encompasses contradictions, exclusivities, opposites and converses. One can love and hate at the same time. One can aspire toward autonomy and desperately wish for dependency at the same moment. The paradigm of suicide is a person who cuts his throat and cries for help at the same time. If you say to such a person "Which do you want to do?" or "Make up your mind," and he has his wits about him, he will respond, "That's precisely the problem, I'm of several minds in the debate within me. I wish to be dead, but I also have fantasies of intervention and rescue." After a natural disaster, in the moments of psychic numbing, this ambivalence is probably not discernible. In a suicidal crisis, it is almost always to be found -- at the very heart of the suicidal crisis. But after a hurricane, or a bombing, or a tornado, the numbing response experienced by the victimized individuals may leave them transiently without ambivalence. They are bereft and, in a sense, psychologically impotent.

What are some of the practical implications of these few points? One is that a variety of kinds of people can do crisis intervention. The second implication is that intervention has to be practical. Crisis intervention is not the best time for fancy psychological interpretations. It's the time for action. One gets other people involved; one mobilizes the significant others, creates action, does practical things.

An illustrative anecdote: Some years ago, at the Los Angeles Suicide Prevention Center, there was an extremely pretty, thirty year old female psychiatric resident. Her patient was an eminent scientist, whose wife had died a couple months before. They had a pact: when one of them died, the other would kill herself/himself. He was very depressed and in the dumps, like a beautiful old ship stopped in the water. He was suicidal and was saving pills, but he was ambivalent enough to telephone the Center. This young physician was assigned to him and she worked with him, doing "her thing." A few weeks later, she discussed him at a staff meeting. (He wasn't there.) She described, in a very matter-of-fact tone, how she had gone up to his apartment (which was a mess), vacuumed it, picked up his papers, did his marketing, did the dishes which lay in the sink; prepared a meal for him, and sort of got him going. And he was better. Some psychiatric residents would have been tempted to sit in their offices and make interpretations about what his wife meant to him, his guilt and his dependency and the loss and so on. But she had gone beyond her training and had given the kind of response that was exactly called for in crisis intervention: activity, concern, action, involvement.

Apropos dependency, it is easy to say banal things about that topic, speaking of "momism," permissiveness and all sorts of things. But I would enjoin you not to include the concept of dependency among your pejorative terms. One hears questions like "Yes, but won't this intensify or prolong his dependency?" In crisis intervention this is nonsense. That might even be the (short-range) goal of the treatment. And even if it isn't, what about it? It's the human condition to be dependent, and in crisis intervention, one can use the dependency, make it a vehicle for helping people by catering to their infantile idiosyncracies. Crisis intervention is not a contest to see who wins. If you make it that way, you ought not be helping them. For how long does one nourish people's dependencies? Until the goals are realized. If one is dealing with a suicidal person who is highly lethal, then the goal is very simple -- to keep that person out of the coroner's office. The usual rules for psychotherapy need to be modified in the service of that goal. In crisis intervention, the response is to the needs of the moment. The goals to roll back the feelings of self anguish, anxiety, general helplessness, affectlessness.

Among the fine things about crisis intervention are the facts that most people can be helped and many individuals have an opportunity to be helpers. Historically, the development of crisis intervention in the last decade, especially with youth helping youth, has led to a democratization of our general psychotherapeutic efforts. I applaud this trend, believing that it offers opportunities for new and more exciting theory-building and that it means that more people will participate in the helping aspects of citizenship.

NOTE: This chapter is an edited version of an extemporaneous presentation given at the opening session of the symposium.

2 : NATURAL SERVICE DELIVERY

Analogies are often helpful in pointing up profound similarities in seemingly diverse processes. Ironically, Dr. Levy provides a disease model analogy to contrast the features of natural and contrived external service delivery mechanisms while later showing that the medical model is limited and inadequate to conceptualize mental health delivery.

The chapter by Dr. Levy emphasizes that naturally occurring mental health services are the most effective and appropriate first line aide. Therefore those interested in the development of mental health services should design that service to make it naturally provided by people already in the phenomenal field of the person in crisis. Later chapters in this book provide illustrations of programs which attempt to take "natural" care givers and add to their helping aramentarium. The move toward the delivery of natural services precludes the professionalization of the service, and denies the utility of the concept of the paraprofessional as a junior grade professional. Dr. Levy would advocate the enhancement of naturally occurring "services" without relabeling them, or trying to incorporate these service delivery agents within the mental health professional guild.

Dr. Levy's analysis of the network television following the death of President Kennedy provides a striking example of a spontaneous, naturally occurring, institutional response to national crisis, which occurred without the input of professional crisis workers. This area may be, however, open to exploration by the creative crisis intervener.

Further analysis of the TV mourning stimulates concern about the forces which determine the kind, scope and form of social crisis intervention. Primary and secondary prevention strategies have a weakness in that they are often anti-democratic. They represent intrusions by "others," (political and appointed powers), who know 'best' how to respond to the needs of a citizen or community in crisis. Proposals for early detection and treatment by in-community, natural forces already have begun to tread on the edge of tyranny.

Dr. Levy makes a strong case for the development of crisis services which are natural and thereby more likely effective. Counterpoint to this presentation can be found in the chapter by McColskey. Perhaps the striking differences between these two positions finds resolution in the fact that both the development of more effective natural mental health services and a corps of highly trained professional crisis workers are all needed to serve different individuals, with different problems. In some sense, the distinction parallels the primary/secondary prevention categorization proposed by Caplan. The "natural" services are in the interest of primary prevention; the highly trained professional can work in secondary prevention and in the enhancement of the "natural" support systems.

THE ROLE OF A NATURAL MENTAL HEALTH SERVICE
DELIVERY SYSTEM IN DEALING WITH BASIC HUMAN PROBLEMS

Leo Levy

University of Illinois at the Medical Center

Chicago, Illinois

For the purposes of this paper, a mental health service delivery system refers to an articulated, planful set of activities aimed at furnishing persons with ameliorative interventions in the cause of reducing their psychological distress. As we currently conceive of this system, it is staffed by professional mental health workers who are not normally a part of the individual's immediate life space. This is to say that the mental health service delivery system with its complement of workers has no other function but to offer mental health services to an individual. To utilize a distinction made in classical Gestalt psychology, the mental health service delivery network exists in the individual's *geographic* environment at all times, but exists in his *phenomenal* environment only at certain times. These periods are characterized by life problems for which the person's normal supportive resources are inadequate and his problem is defined in such a way as to appear relevant to a mental health agency's concerns. Generally, even at this point, it is still necessary for the individual to bring himself to the attention of the agency either directly or via an intermediary. At this point, the agency becomes grafted on, so to speak, to the person's life space or becomes part of his phenomenal environment. The agency performs its function and then recedes into its former background relationship or resumes its status as part of the geographical environment.

A *natural* mental health service delivery system refers to a set of naturally occurring, spontaneously activated mechanisms which are always a part of the individual's phenomenal environment. This network of supportive resources serves similar functions to those described above, but are not manned by mental health professionals and the actors in the system do not generally conceive of their role as primarily related to a mental health function. The family is an instance of this sort, whereas a mental health clinic would serve as an instance of the professional mental health service delivery system.

In order to clarify the model being posed here let us examine two analogous instances having to do with that system we refer to as the human organism. As Walter Cannon pointed out in his important treatise on the human organism (1932), the adaptive functioning of the body may be described in terms of a system of homeostatic mechanisms. One such mechanism is the response of blood components to infection. If the blood stream is invaded by a foreign hostile agent, an immediate, automatic and usually successful chain of defensive reactions transpires. The foreign agent stimulates the production of antibodies which act to neutralize and destroy the agent. This simple recurring drama serves to preserve the life and health of the organism. The mechanism is brought into play spontaneously without the intervention of a sentient contrived external force. Should this mechanism fail as it sometimes does, symptoms of an infection become manifest and we term the person clinically ill. At this point, a physician may be consulted who would in all probability administer an antibiotic to the person. The antibiotic acts as a new externally administered force against the bacterial infection and generally accomplishes the job in which the natural blood protective system had failed. In the first instance we have a prototype for a *natural* service delivery mechanism. In the second instance we have an example of a contrived external service delivery mechanism. Since both accomplish the same end, it would pay us to review the critical differences between the two.

First of all it needs to be noted that the reason why the second system was invoked at all was because of the failure of the first. If the physician's intervention is therapeutic rather than prophylactic, then by definition a disease must exist; in this case an infection. That a disease exists in the organism represents an adaptational failure. Prior to the discovery of antibiotics, our system of medical intervention was largely ineffective and people survived infections because they had good host resistance to disease. People with poor host resistance are repeatedly assaulted by hostile agents and succumb to them. Such individuals may survive only with considerable support from contrived external intervention systems. In other words, a vulnerable organism is at best in a tenuous balance in a hostile environment. When its own internal resources to combat infection are weak, it is closer to death than a stronger organism, though its life may be preserved by repeated external interventions. Furthermore, if the weakness of the defensive resources is genetically transmitted and still allows the organism to survive, one then increases the probability of propagation and the breeding of less disease resistant persons.

Let us now turn to a second analogy dealing with functional defect rather than infection. Suppose a person is deficient in adreno-cortico hormone, and let us suppose further that the adrenal cortex appears structurally sound. Theoretically, the hormone deficiency may be remedied in two ways. The first is to inject cortisol and simply supply the deficient hormone as often as and in amounts required. The second mode of intervention is to administer adreno-cortico-tropic-hormone (ACTH) which has the effect of stimulating the adrenal cortex so that the body supplies itself the deficient hormone. Physicians prefer treatments the effects of which are "physiologic," $i.e.$, strengthen the normal response of the organism. There is good reason for this preference. By supplying adreno-cortico hormone directly, one further reinforces the hypofunctioning of the adrenal cortex; by giving ACTH, one promotes the activity of the gland. The principle is to promote the normal independent functioning of the organism and hopefully free it from dependence on the external support system.

From here I wish to proceed from one system, the human organism, to a more complex superordinate system, that of community, and to contend that the system relationships are analogous. Let us examine the prototypic crisis situation described by Erich Lindemann in 1944, that of bereavement. The principle actor is a human organism, but now conceived as a subsystem of the community system. The crisis situation refers to the experience of the death of a spouse, in this instance death by accident at a young age. The loss is catastrophic and threatens to disable the survivor. The surviving spouse becomes depressed with all the concomitant symptoms; the cumulative effect of which are definitely life threatening.

Spontaneously, and with a certain interesting precision, a series of events transpire which in detail differ from culture to culture, but in form are recognizable everywhere. The survivors of the nuclear family cluster together and interpersonal distance is shortened. Members of the extended family, uncles, aunts, cousins and friends converge on the mourner playing generally nurturing and supportive functions for the disabled survivor. Playing very specific and important roles are a battery of professional persons: a physician, a clergyman, a mortician and perhaps a lawyer. Each plays a specific professional role which one might classify as quintessential to his role in the community. The total process may be characterized as crisis intervention. The players converge on the bereaved, serve a maximal supportive function at the height of the crisis, thus preventing or minimizing disorganization, discontinuity and threat to the survival and well being of the bereaved. As the crisis proceeds towards resolution, and the person begins to reconstitute himself, the entire entourage recedes into its normal background supportive function. The success of the process is measured in terms of the degree to which the survivor is, in fact, reconstituted and independently functioning. Only if this process fails, does the person now find a need for recourse to an external intervention system; in present times, psychiatry or the mental health service delivery system. The fact that this crisis is commonplace and that psychiatrists are rarely consulted on this count attest to the efficacy of the natural service delivery system.

As one will note, the above described *ad hoc* natural service delivery system is manned by other than professional mental health personnel and the system is organic to community process. One might take issue with the assertion that the intervention of the clergyman in this case offering spiritual comfort to a bereaved person is more integral to community process than a psychiatrist offering psychotherapy. In fact, the processes of pastoral guidance and psychotherapy in this instance may even turn out to be highly similar both in technique and content. The argument that one is "natural" and the other "contrived" rests on the inevitability, spontaneity and automaticity of the one intervention as opposed to the other. In the example given earlier of the body's response to infection, the analogue would be the natural generation of antibodies as opposed to the contrived physician intervention with a hyperdermic of penicillin. The fact is that grief is not an automatic cue to a psychiatrist to spontaneously activate himself in regard to the bereaved, whereas for the clergyman it is. Failure of the supportive efforts of the clergyman and other natural interveners to relieve the psychological distress and disorganization is rather the circumstance which leads to the psychiatric referral. It may be that in that brave new distant world acoming, the psychiatrist's intervention in the grief and mourning process may become as inevitable and organic to community process as the clergy's is now. But this is not the case in any culture present or past. Which is not to say that there is anything fixed or immutable about this or any other crisis intervention mechanism now a natural part of community process. As cultures change, so do their support systems. When President John Kennedy was assasinated, the communications media, most notably television, spontaneously became a critical factor in the crisis intervention process. For days, you may recall, a nation of mourners were led through the grief work by almost continuous recounting of the man Kennedy's life, development, the details of his death and finally his interment. There is no question in my mind that a nation of grief stricken persons were guided via this medium through a period of intense psychological distress. Technology changes, community process evolves and thus the form of specific crisis intervention mechanisms change--but not their intent or basic rationale.

The concept of a natural mental health service delivery system appears to be critically implicated in the prevention of mental illness. One significant route to a primary prevention system identifies as many naturally occurring elements of a mental health service delivery system as can be discovered, proceeds to categorize and conceptualize them, support them and if possible improve them. If an appropriate natural service delivery mechanism does not exist, and one could innovate such a mechanism built out of existing elements of communal process, one would be well advised to do so. What I am describing here is a form of social engineering to which behavioral scientists might lend themselves. The analogue given earlier of the physician attempting treatment which results in physiologic efforts, *i.e.*, promotes and enhances the normal response of the organism applies here. The general principle is to enhance and extend the natural service delivery system and keep the contrived external intervention system to a minimum usually reserved for persons for whom the natural service delivery system fails.

Then to speak of a natural mental health service delivery system is to deal with a) community processes spontaneously structured by crisis situations or stressful discontinuities in the life process, and b) persons and institutions outside the traditional mental health sphere which tend to be brought into play as people encounter difficulties in dealing adaptively with problem situations. Such persons are commonly thought of as primary caregivers and include, but are not restricted to, physicians, public health nurses, lawyers, clergymen, public aid caseworkers, teachers, policemen and the institutions which they represent.

In New York City, Morton Bard and his colleagues at the City University have developed what appears to be a promising natural service delivery mechanism based on the use of police as family crisis interveners (Bard & Berkowitz, 1967, 1969). In lower class homes, family disputes frequently result in the police being called. Bard capitalized on this community process by instituting a formal plan of crisis intervention using representative police with special training and ongoing consultation from mental health professionals to respond to family disturbance calls. The program is quite unique and has been evaluated as successful (Bard, 1970). By all reports, the program is acceptable to clients, police interveners and police administrators alike. The service fits the criteria for a natural mental health service delivery system. It is operated by non-mental health professionals and is an extension of an existing spontaneous community process. Other potential natural interveners with regard to family conflict are extended family, friends, public health nurses, clergymen and lawyers. In more relaxed times gone by, the family Doctor might have been turned to and this is undoubtedly still possible in some instances. In the context of this discussion, the family service agency is considered part of the professional mental health service delivery system.

Another common area of psychological distress is the child with behavior problems. The natural contexts for his treatment are the family, the school and the playground. His natural therapists are parents, teachers and playground supervisors. The case for the parent's role in the treatment of the disturbed child has been accepted by mental health professionals from at least the time of Freud. You will recall that in his handling of the case of Little Hans (1909), Freud did not treat the child, but acted as a consultant to his father who applied insights gleaned from discussions with the master. It is standard clinical procedure in child guidance clinics to involve the parents in treatment and more recently family group therapy has become an important treatment vehicle.

Recent developments in behavioral therapy have allowed parents and teachers to become directly involved in the treatment process as lay therapists for disturbed children (Ulrich, Stachnik & Mabry, 1970). It might be noted in passing that the ease with which the "therapist" role may be assigned to parents, teachers or even playmates and school companions in programs of behavioral modification is dictated in part by the relative deemphasis in behavior therapy of the specific character and identity of the therapist. Rather the stress in this mode of therapy is on technique and specifically on the establishment of reinforcement schedules calculated to strengthen or weaken tendencies to behave in a certain fashion. Seen in this light, a Skinner box insofar as it is programmed to carry out certain reinforcement schedules is the instrument for behavior modification, though it is in turn operated by a psychologist. All of which is not to say that a parent or teacher being initially trained via instructions received by a miniature radio transmitter from a professional while working with a child in a natural setting is equivalent to a mechanized reinforcement apparatus. It is rather to indicate that when the therapeutic process is described in terms of discrete operational techniques there is less reliance on complex professional credentials when assigning the role of therapist.

The schools and the playgrounds have not been conventionally thought of as therapeutic settings for the treatment of

behavior problems. This would appear to have less to do with the
the setting than with the perception of the teacher and the playground worker as untrained in psychotherapeutics. These settings,
in fact, are widely emulated by successful clinicians. Reflect
for a moment on some of the better examples of children's treatment centers. Inevitably they resemble a combined family-school-
playground setting more than a mental hospital. Such settings
as Hobb's Project Re-Ed (1966); Warrendale (King, 1967) and the
Orthogenic School (Bettelheim, 1967) spring immediately to mind.
To be sure, the children in these settings are often profoundly
disturbed and thus require workers with at least special training if not a complete professional identity in the mental health
arena. But the bulk of emotional problems of childhood and
adolescence are not of this order and what more felicitous
setting for intervention than where the children naturally aggre-
gate.

In this regard, schools generally sort themselves out into
two categories. The first and traditional role for the school
is as diagnostic and funneling agent. The teacher is usually
felt by mental health professionals and by himself to have the
ability to casefind and then is expected to funnel the disturbed
child into an appropriate agency (*i.e.*, the external service
delivery network). This entails a partial or total extrusion
of the child into an alien system and leaves the teacher and the
school administrator with the comfortable feeling that something
is being done for the child. The possibility that the ideal
treatment milieu and the ideal therapist is being bypassed in
this process has only recently come to be considered. During
the past two decades, mental health consultation with schools
has been widely discussed and recommended by such writers as
Caplan (1970) and Berlin (1956, 1962) to pick two of the more
articulate proponents. With this form of intervention, the disturbed child is not sent to a mental health clinic. Rather a
member of the professional mental health system is used as a
case consultant to the teachers involved with the child. Together, they evolve a treatment plan *in situ* and this plan is
carried forward by the teachers in collaboration possibly with
the guidance counsellor and/or the parents. Here again we see
a natural mental health service delivery system in operation as
an alternative to the use of an external system. Stated otherwise, when teachers extend their function to include systematic
attempts to modify antisocial behavior, maladaptive behavior or
disturbances of normal learning patterns, they are making an extension of an already socially sanctioned and accepted social
role. The teacher, especially with the younger child acts as a
powerful socializing agent and the peer group is a natural therapeutic group as is the family. When the professional mental
health system supports an extension of the school's role in this

fashion, it is developing programs along the lines of primary prevention and one might argue along the lines of secondary prevention as well. The extrusion of the emotionally disturbed child into an external professional mental health system may be viewed as an adaptational failure of the educational subsystem of the community much as the failure of the protective antibodies of the organism to prevent and contain infection may be so viewed.

Similarly playground supervisors, athletic coaches and youth group workers are in an excellent position to intervene constructively in the play situation. One should underscore the manner in which mental health professionals have appropriated this setting for purposes of psychotherapeutic intervention. The accepted mode of psychotherapy with young children is the play situation. With the adolescent, it is often the competitive sport. While it is not, as some exasperated parents might contend, impossible to talk with adolescents, it is certainly easier to do so in the context of a game situation. One mental health center in Chicago in part operates as a pool hall to which adolescents gravitate in the afternoons and evenings. The mental health workers play pool with them and engage in constructive discussions of problems during the game. Here we see the interesting phenomenon of an external service delivery system moving towards a natural one. In fact, considering the identity of the mental health workers involved in this instance--they are somewhat older than the clients but still quite young, indigenous workers who have no formal mental health background-- the two types of systems have become merged. One might even speculate that one significant dimension of future mental health work lies in the direction of the conversion of some contrived external service delivery mechanisms into natural ones. Evidence for this trend is especially impressive from the areas of alcoholism and drug abuse. Alcoholics Anonymous and Synanon are models of treatment in these areas where professional efforts have met with no particularly noteworthy success. These systems exclude professionals as staff and will deal with them only as consultants. A similar trend is in evidence in developing comprehensive community mental health centers, where the style of service delivery is increasingly being built on the indigenous para-professionals called variously mental health workers, psychosocial therapists, etc.

The implication of much of the above discussion leads indirectly to a concept of community organization as a facet of mental health work. Well organized, tightly knit communities where persons sense some control over their destinies appear to produce fewer psychiatric assualties (Levy & Rowitz, 1971). In the light of the discussion of a natural mental health service

delivery system, community articulation and intactness is seen
as a mediating variable in the production of such natural supportive mechanisms. That is, in order to have a natural intervention network as described here, one requires an organized,
viable community. Communities rent by social disorganization
and disruption do not develop and maintain stable mechanisms
which may be characterized as elements of a natural mental
health service delivery network. Thus efforts on the part of
mental health professionals and behavioral scientists to promote integrated community structure are seen as precursive to
the development of stable natural systems of social support.

Isn't this in a larger sense what we have in mind when we
admonish our professional mental health workers to get out of
their offices into the community. Even trends in modes of psychotherapy appear to move in this direction. The weakening of
the taboos against social contact with patients outside the
therapy hour; the lessening insistence on the divorcement of the
therapy hour from the remainder of the person's life and the
trend towards working in natural groupings such as the family
are seen as instances of this kind. And finally, the whole protracted debate over the suitability of the "medical model" as
applied to mental health issues may be viewed in the light of
the issues raised by a natural service delivery system. Maybe
what is being said in several different ways is that psychiatry
is not adequately conceptualized as a medical specialty at
least as medicine is currently practiced. Solutions to human
existential problems do not generally occur in classical psychotherapy, or in traditional mental health institutional frame-
works, but rather occur in the broad stream of natural events
which transpire in that locus that we loosely refer to as community, and it is the failures of this natural system which
then accrue to psychiatry and the professional mental health
system.

NOTE: An earlier version of this paper was prepared for presentation at the sixth annual meeting of the Western Conference on
the Uses of Mental Health Data. October 20-22, 1971. Newport
Beach, California.

REFERENCES

Bard, M. & Berkowitz, B. Training police as specialists in family crisis intervention: A community psychology action program. *Comm. Ment. Health J.* 1967, *3*, 315-317.

Bard, M. & Berkowitz, B. A community psychologic consultation program in police family crisis intervention: preliminary impressions. *Int. J. Soc. Psychiat.* 1969, *XV*, 209-215.

Bard, M. *Training police as specialists in family crisis intervention.* U. S. Govt. Printing Office, Washington, D.C., 1970.

Berlin, I. N. Some learning experiences as a psychiatric consultant in the schools. *Ment. Hyg.* 1956, *XL*, 215-236.

Berlin, I. N. Mental health consultation in the schools as a means of communicating mental health principles. *Amer. Acad. Child Psychiat.* 1962, *1*, 671-679.

Bettelheim, B. *The empty fortress.* New York: The Free Press, 1967.

Cannon, W. B. *The wisdom of the body.* New York: W. W. Norton Co. Inc., 1932.

Caplan, G. *The theory and practice of mental health consultation.* New York: Basic Books Inc., 1970.

Freud, S. Analysis of a phobia in a five year old boy in *Collected Papers,* London: Hogarth Press, 1957, Volume III, 149-289.

Hobbs, N. Helping disturbed children: psychological and ecological strategies. *Amer. Psychol.* 1966, *21*, 1105-1115.

King, A. *Warrendale.* New York: Grove Press, Inc., 1967.

Levy, L. & Rowitz, L. Ecological attributes of high and low rate mental hospital utilization areas in Chicago. *Social Psychiatry,* 1971, *6*, 20-28.

Lindemann, E. Symptomatology and management of acute grief. *Amer. J. Psychiat.* 1944, *101*, 111-148.

Ulrich, R., Stachnik, T. & Mabry, J. (Eds.) *Control of human behavior.* Volume II, Scott, Foresman and Co., 1970.

3: CRISIS ASSESSMENT AND REDUCTION

Crisis can be defined essentially as the result of a temporary loss of behavioral control occurring typically in transitional periods in which normal support sources are weakened or absent. Dr. Korner distinguishes between 'exhaustion' and 'shock' crises. The former represents a crises developing following a prolonged attempt to deal with overwhelming problems. The latter refers to crises developing consequent to a major precipitating event. Intervention technique should be appropriate to the type of crisis.

The effective diagnosis of a person's strength and capabilities for ongoing functioning is an essential aspect of crisis intervention. In a parallel to the mental status examination used to evaluate admitting patients, Dr. Korner suggests that the crisis worker evaluate the coping potential of the individual by reviewing the availability of six major sources of support including 1) intellectual operations, 2) friends and neighbors, 3) free emotional motivating forces such as anger, 4) hope, 5) the motivation to help oneself and, 6) the individual's personal contribution to the crisis.

The person suffering from reduced functioning, as a result of emotional overloading in a shock crisis, requires new channels of communication; forceful impingement of the external environment on an individual may facilitate improvement. Dr. Korner sees it as essential to combat passivity and to use any available motivational forces to help the person regain a feeling of competence and to prevent the person's acceptance of the sick and helpless role. Mastery can be enhanced by catharsis, environmental and personal support and increased use of rational logical thinking. Feelings of weakness and insecurity result from the realization of failure to effectively manage the crisis. The crisis worker can push the client toward competent, effective responses which will provide improved chances of successful mastery of future crisis by avoiding the negative personal attitudinal consequences of failure.

The two examples illustrating Dr. Korner's concept of intervention are likely to stir controversy. In each case, Dr. Korner resorts to active, dramatic intervention, providing literal impingement of the intervenor into the life of the person in crisis; these techniques are foreign to most traditional clinical training, and most professionals find them difficult to implement.

We think this is a stimulating chapter which should be thoughtfully considered by trainers and practitioners in the crisis intervention area. We also welcome Dr. Korner's call for improved models and theory as well as elaboration of effective intervention techniques. For Dr. Korner, crisis intervention means something quite different than short term individual psychotherapy.

CRISIS REDUCTION AND THE PSYCHOLOGICAL CONSULTANT

I. N. Korner

University of Wisconsin-Green Bay

Personal crises occur in every individual's life. Most of these the individual copes with by drawing upon his own resources, in the privacy of his loneliness; no one ever hears or knows about them. Severe crisis, however, may present baffling and confusing conditions with which common sense and prior experience have not equipped the individual to cope. This is particularly likely to occur in those institutions where large numbers of individuals must meet crisis conditions without the customary protection and aid of friends and families: the armed services; college, especially the freshman and senior years; the "first job"; and the beginning years of marriage. When crisis are precipitated in such contexts, where support and help from everyday associates is inadequate or nonexistent, the skills of the psychologist-consultant often come into play, with long-lasting consequences for the individual undergoing the crisis condition. For success in overcoming a crisis adds to individual strength and coping potential, while failure may permanently undermine this potential.

When a psychologist-clinician faces an individual he has never seen before in the midst of an acute crisis condition, he encounters new and unfamiliar problems. He is probably accustomed to evaluating suffering individuals on a theoretical health-illness continuum, diagnosing and making plans to move the individual in the direction of health. To replace discomfort and illness with comfort, well-being, and vitality, is his primary task, and time is ordinarily not of the essence. However, in the role of psychologist-consultant, a radically different perspective is called for. His function now is to reduce the proportion of the crisis to the point where the individual is enabled to cope with it on his own, and in doing so time *is* of the very essence, for a crisis is by definition a situation in which events are occurring with overwhelming rapidity. Thus the psychologist must relegate his usual concern for theoretical criteria of discomfort, health, and illness, and treatment needs to a subordinate position in deference to the primary goal, which is to create constructive change in the individual's condition as rapidly as possible. Deterioration of the capacity to cope must be halted and reversed in an effective crisis consultation. Only then can the traditional functions and purposes of the psychologist reemerge as primary concerns.

However, even though "diagnosis" is a superfluous activity in crisis intervention, the consultant still must evaluate the precipitating circumstances of the crisis and the coping potential of the individual if his help is to be of value, and this must be done within some frame of reference. This paper addresses itself to the development of such a framework, with the goal of identifying the key dynamics influencing crisis situations and focusing the consultant's attention upon them without the distinction of standard theoretical (psychoanalytic) formulations which usually require a certain modicum of intellectual leisure for fruitful application. While the discussion which follows is not inconsistent with clinical theories, it ignores their finer points and concentrates upon those aspects of the individual's condition most critical to quick and effective crisis consultation.

First, what is the psychological nature of a crisis? A fact of central significance is that some of the functions which control behavior have been temporarily lost (not permanently lost; in the latter case the situation would be described not as a crisis, but as a collapse). In a crisis, the tacit assumption is made that the situation is reversible. One response to crisis may be a severe reduction in coping ability; environmental conditions have attained and/or made inoperative the habitual methods for dealing with discomfort, feelings of insecurity, anxiety and fear, etc. When these cannot be contained any longer, a level of disorganization is incurred which is often called "panic," wherein the intellectual control mechanism has become inoperative under an onslaught of unchecked, unintegrated emotional stimuli. The individual is unable to use cognitive elements (arguments, deliberations, judgments, perspectives of others) to control, check or reduce the magnitude and affects of his emotional reactions. He has no further means of defense at his disposition--temporarily coping has ceased, or nearly ceased.

An important differentiation must be introduced at this point. There are two different etiological processes which precipitate crisis, each prognosticating different outcomes and, therefore, demanding different methods of handling by the consultant. The individual may have coped effectively for some time under prolonged conditions of emergency, when he suddenly reaches the point of exhaustion. There is simply not enough strength left to sustain the available coping resources, and the result is a quasi-ungluing of the total coping structure. This state will be referred to as the "exhaustion crisis." A crisis, on the other hand, may result when a sudden change in the environment creates an explosive release of emotions which overwhelm the available coping mechanism. An individual who can deal with adversity provided he has the time to assimilate the impact may be unable to do so then events occur rapidly and without forewarning; he goes into emotional shock. This state will be referred to as "shock crisis."

There is still another source of crisis which may be inextricably linked with the other two. Rather than being the "victim," the individual may in fact be the originator of his own crisis, which was precipitated in the service of his needs to control his environment. This condition is familiar to the experienced psychologist and does not represent a *bona fide* crisis condition. This situation will be considered here only as a possible factor in any crisis; it is referred to as "the purposive element of crisis."

The term "coping potential" has been used several times in the discussion thus far, and it is a concept of key significance. The crisis itself represents a reduction in the ability to cope. Successful coping, in turn, represents the ability to ward off by all means, the occurrence of crisis condition. Once a crisis condition has set in it is the consultant's task to revive and strengthen coping abilities. The clinician will recognize that "coping potential" in this context bears a clear relation to the familiar concepts of ego strength and ego resources as used in therapeutic assessments. Considerable controversy shrouds the notion of ego strength. It is difficult to define, and even more difficult to translate into behavioral equivalents. The substitution of the term "coping potential" is not designed to replace one vague abstraction with another equally vague; it is rather an attempt to link the overall concept of the rational, reality-contact functions of the personality as directly as possible with observable action patterns. "Coping potential" is defined here as those behavioral functions enabling the organism to maintain himself in his environment continuously and preserving his ability to do so. The term "coping mechanism" should be used only when a preferably describable set of events which predictably would lead to disorganization, conflict, reduction and/or loss of adjustment ability, is reacted to with behavior patterns aimed at influencing the internal and external environment in such a way as to insure an avoidance of or an elimination of a developing and/or progressing crisis condition. (The individual, for example, reacts to an external structure with fear which interferes with his perceptual-organizational ability which in turn prevents further investigation of the stimulus. This provokes more fear, and so in an ever widening vicious circle of events a crisis is in the making. The individual capacity to break the spiral of developments and incur the return of his problem-solving capabilities represents his coping abilities.)

Depending upon the availability and efficacy of the coping potential, there are six areas the consultant needs to evaluate:

1. *How many of the intellectual functions are capable of minimally adequate operation?*

A request for an account of the events preceding the crisis will provide an answer. If the individual can give an account, if upon further questioning he is able to provide details, if he can be made to consult his memory, the intellectual components of his coping mechanism can be considered intact. The consultant may want to check further. Can the individual use his intellectual resources for self-inspection, self-organization? The consultant may test this by giving a small explanatory interpretation. If the individual registers the explanation, and possibly accepts its validity or finds it helpful, "insight" may be available as a possible source for controlling the crisis situation.

2. *What interpersonal assets are available?*

A discussion of the "significant people" in the individual's environment will yield this information. Each time the individual mentions a significant person, the consultant should ask: "Would you like to see this person now? Would his or her presence be helpful? Can we call in this person to talk with us? (This should be done casually and within the context of the conversation.) The consultant also may use subtle suggestions or questions about what help he himself might contribute; can the individual use the relationship offered? Does he respond to a personal comment, to a warm smile, to a gesture of encouragement? If the individual responds to his interviewer, if he finds the presence of significant people helpful, he is able to use human resources and interpersonal relationships, and this coping resource may be available.

3. *What emotional resources are available to contain the disorganization?*

Though anxiety, fear and discomfort may be rampant, rarely are *all* emotions out of control. The individual may be able to verbalize freely about anger, affection, or other emotions which are still under control. Emotional reactions must be carefully evaluated and can be used to advantage toward the reduction of the crisis condition. Anger, to use an example, may be used to advantage to bind, push back, repress, deny, or rationalize conditions which are generating the fear and discomfort. Anger can be used to control other emotions, and may serve as a successful antidote to generalized feelings of helplessness.

A second line of inquiry pertains to those feelings which are directly responsible for the crisis condition. This investigation demands some of the skills of the clinically trained individual. It is helplessness, fear, anxiety, unexpressed rage, deep personal hurt, loss of an interpersonal relationship, or loss of hope which accounts for suddenly manifested lack of organization and control. If these can be brought to open expression, perhaps the individual will be helped; however, if even the smallest contact with the untamed effects leads to greater disorganization, it must be avoided. The perusal of the field of emotions should be handled with care unless the consultant is experienced in this task.

4. *What are the dimensions of the hope structure? Can it be activated for the purpose of control?*

In an earlier article (Korner, 1970), this was discussed in considerable detail. The sudden loss and/or destruction of something hoped for can produce crisis conditions. Any hope structure, can be said to have two main components. The first, is an affect-laden, belief like component, the second, is a rationale for considering that the desired occurrence has a high probability. The first component represents the *raison d'etre* for the hope; the second component gives the first a logical framework. Hopes represent important coping mechanisms. The destruction of either the first or the second component can severely upset an individual's psychological equilibrium. Hope can be reinstated, replaced, or compensated for which concomitantly alleviates the crisis condition.

5. *How much motivation does the individual have to help himself?*

Of all the questions, this is the one most difficult to answer. The individual can often be asked directly whether he feels able to help in his own recovery by performing certain tasks; the following questions represent a possible sequence of demands. His responses may be very useful in assessing his participation potential.

Can you help us by trying to think about what happened that you started feeling this way?

Can you help us by telling us how you feel just now?

Can you help us by calling the person who is involved?

Can you help us by going back into this situation to find out if things are really the way you think they are?

Can you help us, you and me, by trying harder to remember?

When do you think you will be able to handle this on your own?

Can you take care of yourself now?

When will you be able to take care of yourself?

6. *To what degree has the individual himself created or aggravated the crisis condition?*

This can only be established usually at the end of an assessment and only if sufficient background information has been obtained. The individual who displays a considerable flair for dramatic or histrionic behavior, or who attempts to impress subtly or crudely, upon the consultant his own tragedy and the tragedy of the situation, is liable to fall into this group. It presents the consultant with the necessity for caution with his empathy and attempts at support.

Answers to the above six questions should be taken with reservations. They should be used only to form an hypothesis concerning the individual's state of readiness to act on his own behalf. The six points discussed presume that the individual is able to communicate verbally. This is not always the case. Extreme and severe crisis conditions provide rather frightening encounters for the consultant. The individual may be crying convulsively or mute, his glance glazed, his response to direction minimal; he may be unaware of people, sealed off from communications. For prolonged periods there may be but rudimentary intellectual and emotional control, with greatly reduced interpersonal awareness and capacity to respond. Extreme crisis represent grave psychological conditions which the consultant must attack immediately. Bringing the individual into some form of contact with his environment is the consultant's first and immediate task. The means available are rather primitive, but quite effective; the theoretical assumptions are few and simple. They are the following:

1. Personality integration is reduced due to emotional overloading.
2. Mechanisms for reduction of the emotional hypertension are

inoperative.
3. The emotional tension level can be reduced only by opening
   channels of communication toward the environment.
4. As the individual is not able to move toward the environment, the environment has to penetrate to the individual.

Ancient means for achieving this are yelling, slapping, in-
flicting physical shocks to the body in extreme cases, punching
and hair-pulling. The Edwardian Age used for the control of
female crisis behavior the application of smelling salts. Also
effective is simply to talk to the individual. "Talk" represents a social demand which more often than not will prove a
stimulus hard to resist. It is good practice to make the individual angry, provided anger is not the source of disorganization. Anger is a tonic, it instills motivation to move toward
the offending object, it creates action. It sets emotions into
motion toward the environment, thus working in the direction of
crisis reduction. Reduced intellectual control can be improved
by making demands of the individual. The individual needs to
be stirred up, his passivity must be combatted.

All these are strange behaviors indeed for a consultant
trained in the clinical tradition. The approach to psychological suffering favored by the customary psychotherapeutic practice emphasizes warmth, compassion, empathy, concern and kind-
ness. This approach may be unwise in a crisis condition; in
fact, it may do more harm than good, by encouraging the individual to remain in the passive comfort of inactivity. In a severe
crisis condition, the consultant may have to force himself to
act against his own professional posture. Questions may have to
be asked aggressively, sometimes abrasively. When the answers
are unintelligible he has to insist: "Speak clearly! No, I *don't*
understand what you mean." "I cannot understand you; can you
talk clearly and make sense?" etc. Aggressiveness or emotional
neutrality,frequently will lead, as discussed above to counter-
actions which channel the individual's emotions outward and
toward discharge. An aggressive-abrasive attitude by the consultant represents an emergency tool to be used with considerable care and discretion and,if successful, should be replaced
immediately by an attitude of understanding and emphatic participation.

Once the individual's intellect is beginning to exert some
form of control over the internal and then gradually upon his
external environment, the result of evaluations can be used. If
emotional expression can be instituted and interpersonal contacts activated even to a minimal degree, it can be assumed that
the crisis will subside provided favorable conditions are maintained. These may include the company of significant and close
people, sleep, food, engagement in activity, etc.

If in spite of efforts the individual refuses to engage in interpersonal contacts and/or is unable to gain control over his emotional diffuseness, if his inability to regain emotional discharge persists, the situation is critical. It may not be amenable to crisis abatement techniques; it may not represent an ordinary crisis situation. Earlier the term "exhaustion crisis" was coined to describe a situation where the tools and techniques of coping with prolonged stresses led to a sudden break, an abrupt cessation of efforts due to the exhaustion of the ultimate reserves of the individual. Efforts to draw the individual back to the environment are met less with resistance, than with apathy, impotence and indifference. There is an air of ultra-resignation, of lethargic "I don't care any more" which may serve as a guide to the correct assessment of the situation. With "exhausted" individuals an active attempt to push and pull, to reverse the exhaustion into activity, may produce the opposite of the desired effects. The pressure represents a further environmental demand which the individual simply is unable to meet. Crisis counteracting measures discussed in this paper are not to be used with 'exhaustion' situations. The answer to exhaustion is slow replenishment in a benign environment to which the individual must be referred at the earliest. Having diagnosed an exhaustion state, further activities by the consultant cease.

Any refusal by the individual to resume contact with the environment poses a dilemma to the psychologist-consultant, who is aware that the crisis must find a speedy solution. He is greatly concerned about the choices the individual is about to make. The psychologist-consultant is never neutral in regard to the outcome of the crisis. Of the many solutions the individual can choose to terminate the crisis, the consultant prefers some and is opposed to others. The consultant opposes the solution in which the individual chooses the sick role as a method to terminate the crisis condition. Any individual in crisis makes the social environment respond with concern and care. At times individuals, particularly those under stress, crave the concern, the interest, the solicitude which the crisis has created. They may want to continue in the situation of emergency. Too much or too long a prepetuation of the concern and care situation may prove to be a powerful invitation to the adoption of the "sick role." The adoption of the "sick role" by the individual is an undesirable solution to a crisis. To individuals moving in that direction, the consultant must refuse extra attention and concern. The psychologist cannot afford, in the interest of the individual, to be warm and considerate, supportive and helpful, without further deliberations as to their effect. He must maintain a friendly, neutral attitude and extend but moderate sympathy.

The resumption of control is slow and painful, to be accomplished in due time and sequence. Hesitance to resume the burden of control may be but a preliminary to resumption; pressure at this moment could have adverse affects upon the process of recovery. The individual groping for mastery needs thoughtful, sympathetic often non-verbal companionship and support. Whether to extend support, to what degree and with what assistance remains the decision of the consultant. It must be synchronized with the individual and his needs and the style of his recovery. The consultant often faces painful dilemmas and uncomfortably weighty choices.

The individual in order to master a crisis condition needs to accomplish the following tasks:

1. He has to regain mastery over the unintegrated affects. He can accomplish this by three main methods: *First* by letting the emotions circulate freely outward into the environment; in due time, they may spend themselves. A prolonged crying spell often accomplishes this. *Second,* by perceiving the presence of others as supportive. This may provide the margin of safety and courage from which emerges the decision to resume coping attempts. The presence of another individual who provides security, sympathy, and companionship reduces the level of anxiety and therefore can accomplish a reduction of the intensity of the rampant emotions. This provides an opportunity for the submerged coping mechanisms to re-emerge. *Third,* the increase in the use of the cognitive, rational tools at the individual's disposition will decrease the chaos and re-establish control. Facts, events, opinions, can be presented to the individual which he can use to develop thoughts and ideas which in turn can block, surround, or deactivate affective masses.

To use an example, the individual may have incurred a vital loss of a personal bond. The psychologist has the alternative mentioned above. He may make comments which encourage the expression of feelings ("This hurt you more than you could tolerate," "There also must have been some anger in what you felt," etc.) The second alternative sees the consultant assume an attitude of friendly but silent waiting, keeping company. Or he may want to introduce elements of reasoning into the individual's turmoil: "What do you think made him do it at this time?" What do you object most to about the way she did it?" "What would have helped you most if you had known more beforehand?" The choice of emotional expression over the strengthening of cognitive elements is best based on assessments, but more often is a matter of intuition. It becomes quickly apparent whether the choice was the right one, and errors must be corrected immediately without pride or prejudice.

2. Having gained mastery, the individual has to deal with a secondary problem, his own concern and apprehension over his reactions to the crisis which may well leave him with considerable consternation, apprehension, anxiety and discomfort. To have given way to panic leaves large residues of insecurity in all individuals who experience it. The psychologist-consultant must bring this issue up for discussion and explanation, so the individual may be helped to integrate the crisis experience rather than to reject it. It may be helpful to discuss not only the person's feelings about his behavior, but its possible social implications; the consultant may ask questions, explain, and perhaps give advice with the goal of building understanding and resistance.

3. Even under the best conditions of recovery, the individual needs some assurance against reoccurrence of crisis conditions. Some form of potential support must be arranged. In the absence of family and close friends, the psychologist must make himself available. This must be handled with subtlety or it may be misinterpreted by the individual as an indication that the psychologist-consultant considers a potential reoccurrence of the crisis condition a possibility. The offer of support is a two-edged sword. To one person it is an offer of strength to be leaned on with pleasure, to another it represents the consultant's doubts about the individual's ability to stand on his own feet. The psychologist must make sure that his concern is properly understood, not as a doubt, but as a useful offer of comfort. This can be accomplished by offering the individual not an appointment but an opportunity to "chat" upon his request and pleasure.

The activities of the crisis specialist at this point are terminated, but the concern for the well-being of the individual transcends limitations imposed by professional specialization. What further care does the individual need subsequent to the return of his pre-crisis state? If the crisis was the result of rather extraordinary, rarely recurring event, no further care needs to be suggested. If the individual appears to have given away under relatively little environmental pressure, referral for further study is indicated.

Following are descriptions of two successful reductions of acute crisis experiences which may serve to illustrate how the framework outlined above applies in practice.

1. Carol, a woman in her early twenties living alone in a simple apartment in a lower middle class neighborhood, was found by her neighbors in a state of shocked muteness. She was sitting stiffly in a chair and appeared not to have moved for hours. She stared into space and took no cognizance of the

events in her environment. The neighbors could give little information beyond the fact that they had become concerned when
Carol had not collected the milk and the paper. They had knock-
ed on the door, and when no answer came forth had gained entry
with a passkey Her condition was unchanged when the consultant
arrived. He turned to Carol and started asking questions, repeating the same questions again and again in an ever louder
voice which ended up in shouting. At the same time he shook her
gently by her shoulder. It was when the consultant had nearly
given up hope and turned away that Carol ceased to stare blankly
and looked at him with something resembling absentmindedness.
The talking and shaking was continued with vigor. She suddenly
looked fully at the worker and commenced to whimper. Holding
her unresponsive hands, the consultant continued to talk with
little memory of what he said. The whimpering changed into crying which became progressively more violent as the physical rigidity slowly subsided. There still was no verbal communication.
The worker continued to talk to her. Her crying became a bit in-
human, like the sounds of an animal in pain. She contracted
physically and started to shake violently. The worker put his
arm around her and tried to comfort her. When the sobbing started to subside, the whole previous sequence having lasted for
about half an hour, the consultant commenced to ask questions in
a rather determined and examining way. ("Tell me what happened,
you have to tell me what happened.") Still turning away, and
interrupted by bouts of crying and sobbing she told her story.

    She had come to the city from a small town. She had ob-
tained a position as a secretary. She had met a "fascinating"
man on the job. They had an affair. Her first. She was terribly happy that "this experienced man of the world had found
her interesting and worthy of his love." They had discussed
getting married in the near future and she had made elaborate
plans for a wedding, an event second to none to a girl with her
kind of up-bringing. But she had received the previous evening
a letter from her fiancee, telling her rather crudely that he did
not want to see her any more and not to bother with any attempts
to contact him. She tried to reach him by phone all evening and
finally succeeded after midnight. Again, he told her curtly not
to bother him. She had no memory of any events subsequent to the
phone conversation, prior to talking with the consultant. She
declined an offer for help, but quite obviously wanted to talk.
She reacted with silence to the consultant's suggestion that the
telephone conversation seemed to have shocked her. She finally
commented: "It was not the telephone conversation, it was the
letter. It hit me really only after I had tried to reach him.
When he said it again on the phone I knew the letter was true."

    At this point the worker concluded that her intellectual
functions were operating fully and that her potential for using

interpersonal resources was good. He next suggested that she
might be feeling anger. She denied any emotions except surprise
and hurt. She defended the man's actions, because after all she
"knew all the time that it could not last." The worker concluded that her affective mobility was still quite restricted and
that he needed to know whether this represented part of the
crisis or was part of her permanent personality organization.
He brought the discussion to other shocks she had experienced in
the past, when it appeared that she had led a rather sheltered
existence. In the discussion of her relationships to the significant people of her environment, she revealed a pattern of
well-controlled expression of anger and affection. It therefore
appeared that she was still under considerable emotional pressure,
unable, as yet, to function with her customary emotional freedom.
The worker proceeded to discuss the nature of a crisis and found
her listening as well as taking part in the conversation.

The consultant tried to probe for the nature of her hope
structure. (This must be a blow to your hope. Do you feel you
will find someone to marry like the one who disappointed you?
Do you hope to love again?) Her answers revealed that her hope
structure was not involved in the crisis. She had not "hoped"
to marry the man, it has been a reality, a certainty as far as
she was concerned. She felt terribly disappointed about the
facts of her broken relationship. She declined to think about
the future but she felt no "hope" nor did she seem to want any
"hope" that the relationship would be reconstructed.

She gave no impression that she had either added to or obtained any kind of satisfaction from her state of crisis.

The consultant now faced the difficult decision of advising
her to return home to a benign environment conducive to healing
psychological injuries, trusting her powers of self-recovery, or
arranging for a speedy referral to a treatment facility. He remembered a comment she had made earlier when she expressed concern about being absent from her job. With some trepidation,
the worker decided to trust her strength and power of recovery.
He suggested and Carol agreed to, returning to work for the
afternoon. ("The man" did not work there any more.) She accepted the suggestion of professional help which was not described
as psychotherapy but rather as "talking to someone who has had
lots of experience with people who are in the process of psychological mending." She agreed to call the consultant in the
evening. He arranged an appointment for the next day with a
community agency. Carol was interviewed six months later, and
the recovery appeared complete, though the rather painful lesson
in living had a profound after-affect and was still observable.
She had not dated and was not thinking of doing so. She viewed
her future as offering her professional advancement and related

to it the chance to travel. She had given up the notion of marriage and settling in her home town or not too far away from it.
She gave the impression of being somewhat rootless and lacking
in aims.

II. The second example is drawn from the college environment, a
place where crisis is a frequent occurrence. Often it is handled *in situ* by friends, classmates, or residence-hall mates.
Only where the latter become frightened or feel unequal to the
task is a mental health agent called on for help. As the principles of evaluation and crisis-counteraction are the same as in
the previously presented example, this account will be limited
to the basic events.

The consultant was called in by a group of six young men
sharing an apartment. The youngest member of the group, Jim,
was in great distress. He had been tense for a number of days;
his roommate reported that Jim had slept little and badly. The
night before, Jim had been out, drinking heavily. He had returned in the early morning hours, gone to bed, and stayed there
for the day. He had not participated in any of the customary
activities, he had sat alone in the room, fending off gruffly
all attempts to communicate. All this was highly uncharacter-
istic of Jim's usual behavior which could be described best as
square, friendly, and considerate.

The consultant entered Jim's room and was introduced by a
fellow student. Jim rebuked all efforts of the consultant to
open a conversation and finally yelled, "Leave me alone!" After
some thought, the consultant asked, "Would it bother you if I
just stayed quietly for a while?" Jim answered, "Suit yourself."
(The presence of a silent "other person" represents a strong
social stimulus.) After some time spent in active silence, Jim
said curtly, "So what good does this do?" The consultant responded in low key, "not being alone always helps." In the ensuing conversation, Jim tried to play down his difficulties,
tried to explain away his behavior by pointing to the stress of
college life in general. Only gradually, helped by occasional
questions, did he reveal that he had moved six weeks ago from
the residence hall, where he was doing well, into the shared
apartment. He did so because he wanted to try living off campus,
and he had been invited to move in by a friend. He came from a
middle-class family, the younger of two boys. He appeared to
love his family and considered his father and brother his closest friends. Going to the college and living in the residence
hall was not easy, but not too difficult either. He had suffered from, but adjusted to, loneliness. But since moving to
the apartment, he had felt less and less capable to deal with
what he called his *irritations*. He acknowledged his perturbance

but could not accept and/or understand that his "annoyances" could be related to his present total upset. Encouraged to talk about the "annoyances," the dam burst open: Inconsiderations from the others; his things were not respected; people did not take care of their responsibilities; people did not talk out their problems, irritations, or complaints in a problem solving way," on and on. The consultant concluded that Jim came from an unusually harmonious, isolated background with great and elegant skills in intimate human relationships. These social skills were of little avail to him in the rough and tumble of his new micro-society. He was unable to transmit his messages, he was equally unable to hear messages given to him in an unfamiliar style and language. His personality was unsuited to cope with the large masses of frustration, anger, and bewilderment this gave rise to. He felt himself trapped between his tempestuous emotional reactions which in their intensity were unfamiliar to him, and his inability to solve his problems with his available social skills. Jim: "I just cannot go and tell these guys that they are a rude, crude bunch of animals. I also know it is not their problem; they are doing all right among themselves. It is my problem so how can I tell them? I tried and they laughted and told me to take it easy. I don't want to just leave and face all the questions of what happened." Jim felt trapped. The consultant suggested that with all the fellows being at home and greatly concerned about his well-being, a group conversation might be profitable. He, the consultant, could stay and help the thing go smoothly. He also could perhaps help explain, if necessary, Jim's problem to the others. The proposal was reluctantly accepted by Jim, but received enthusiastically by his mates, who were genuinely unaware of the nature of Jim's problems. The seminar lasted for a number of hours. Jim's "trap" led to a general discussion of human relations, transgressing by far the original intent of the discussion. Jim was helped. He stayed for the rest of the year in the apartment, seemingly with good and profitable effects. He did, though, move back to the residence hall the next year.

The foregoing cases illustrate that the application of clinical theory for the purpose of reinstituting coping behavior is neither necessary nor desirable, since the occurrence of a crisis does not indicate that the affected individual is prone to psychological deficiency, illness, or breakdown. Crisis is usually the result of aggravated, precipitated living conditions and presents in most instances a choice situation leading either to recovery of normal coping or to further retreat from such recovery with potential long-term weakening of the coping structure. The goal of crisis intervention is to facilitate immediate recovery; in view of the quantity of crisis-producing situations this society has spawned, success in this endeavor would be a preventive mental health measure of no mean proportions.

More resources need to be directed into the development of theoretical formulations and research methodologies which will increase our understanding of the theory and practice of crisis intervention.

REFERENCES

Korner, I. N.   Hope as a method of coping. *Journal of Counseling and Clinical Psychology*, 1970, *34*, 134-139.

III: PERSONNEL AND TRAINING

The professional/paraprofessional argument continues: are non-professionals competent to handle individuals in intense crisis when actions will have profound effects on the future adjustment of the individual? We provide no answer to this question, but by way of the McColskey tract hope to focus the issue more sharply.

Since non-professionals in crisis intervention proliferate the presentations by Sebolt, Stern and Berman all should be helpful in the operation, management and evaluation of emergency mental health services.

Though underrepresented in terms of pages, we see the development of useful, constructive research strategies essential to the development of a viable, stable "science" of practice in crisis intervention. Several of the contributing authors have shown how research can be integrated into the development of a new program, and Bleach has suggested ways in which research can be grafted into an operation with a minimum of disruption. Further development of quasiexperimental methods aimed at answering the important questions is essential for the maturing of this area.

4: PROFESSIONAL CRISIS COUNSELING

This chapter by Dr. Ann McColskey speaks directly to some
of the issues raised in the introductory chapter. Specifically,
Dr. McColskey treats the question of whether professionals and
non-professional crisis workers can function to similar effects.
She concludes that this is not the case. In essence, she argues
that the clinical skills and career commitments of the professional are necessary for the establishment of truly effective
and stable crisis centers. She further specifies that centers
in which professionals are paid for their services most closely
approximate the ideal model, offering a program in Florida as
an exemplar.

Of particular interest in Dr. McColskey's paper is her
treatment of the cost-benefit aspects of professionally staffed
crisis centers. The use of lay staff in crisis centers seems to
offer an economy, both in terms of financial and manpower resources. Dr. McColskey suggests, however, that the training
costs, administrative problems, and turnover rate for non-professionals at least partially offset the advantages of such
staffing. The center which she cites as a model conserves resources by giving professional staffers compensatory time from
their other duties in a community mental health center as repayment for their work in crisis counseling. This approach does
not reduce the actual cost of professional staffing, but does
"hide" the expense under existing funding allotments. The viability of a time repayment arrangement depends upon the possibi-
ity of having the professional perform his full allotted responsibilities, outside of crisis work, in less than the time
budgeted for the tasks. Thus, the proposed model actually ex-
pands manpower resources by requiring the professional to pro-
 ide increased amounts of service in a fixed time; if he cannot
do so, the model fails. The plan might apparently succeed, however, at the unnoticed cost of a reduction in the amount of
necessary but unappealing work completed.

Another issue relates to the actual, as opposed to the
ascribed, skills of different types of crisis center personnel.
Dr. McColskey's preference for professional workers seems to

rest on two assumptions. First, it is assumed that tradition-
ally trained mental health workers actually possess the basic
skills appropriate for crisis work. Second, it is assumed that
non-professional workers do not offer actual advantages over
more highly trained personnel. Later chapters in this book,
particularly those of Sebolt and Jaffe, raise serious questions
about the validity of these assumptions. It may yet be that the
enthusiasm, lack of theoretical bias, and lesser role conflict
of the non-professional actually give him advantages over the
professional worker. Whatever, Dr. McColskey's chapter clearly
provides some balance of perspective in a field whose non-pro-
fessionalism has been more the rule than the exception.

MODELS OF CRISIS INTERVENTION: THE CRISIS COUNSELING MODEL

Ann S. McColskey

Clinical Psychologist, Pensacola, Florida

In considering "crisis intervention" models, one is met with a bewildering variety of examples, serving a variety of purposes and value systems under that broad rubric. If, however, the various models are arrayed along two dimensions, a professional/lay dimension and a volunteer/compensated dimension, some order is introduced into the universe and rational comparisons can more readily be made. These distinctions are not always clearly rendered--"volunteer," *e.g.*, is sometimes loosely contrasted with "professional," in discussion of "crisis intervention" models, as if these were antonyms, and it should be clearly kept in mind that they are not and that two orthogonal, unrelated dimensions are involved. Volunteers may be and are professionals, subprofessionals, preprofessionals, and paraprofessionals--every variant of trained worker as well as lay helpers, in "crisis intervention" programs.

The professional/lay dimension is of course the primary dimension, insofar as the character of a particular "crisis intervention" program is concerned; the volunteer/compensated dimension is a secondary, utilitarian dimension. There are other secondary descriptive continua that can be considered in classifying "crisis intervention" programs: a continuum of breadth or comprehensiveness of services, for one, ranging from narrowly-conceived, brief, superficial intervention in suicidal crises (limited to rescue efforts and/or referrals to other agencies) or stopgap drug therapy, at one end of the continuum, to broad-spectrum crisis management and continued psychotherapeutic care at the other end, and, for another, a continuum of directness/indirectness (of interventive efforts), ranging from direct, face-to-face contacts to indirect phone intervention.

If "crisis intervention" models are first arrayed along the primary, professional/lay dimension and dichotomized as either professional or non-professional in general character, the other three dimensions can be utilized to limn out secondary differen-

tiating characteristics of programs of each type, to facilitate
comparison and choice.

NON-PROFESSIONAL "CRISIS INTERVENTION" PROGRAMS

Considering first, then, the broad category of non-professional "crisis intervention" programs, it may be stated that,
from a theoretical point-of-view, the concept of a program of
this type represents a contradiction in terms--that there is no
logical justification for an emergency mental health service
manned by unskilled workers. Logically, if professional training in one of the mental health disciplines is considered a requisite for management of psychological problems, then adjustmental crises or acute problems demand the utmost--not the
least--in expertise. Conceptually, the notion of using untrained persons to manage crisis-reactions is as illogical and hazardous as attempting to stem a massive hemorrhage with a band-aid.

"Suicide Prevention" Programs

The argument has been advanced (McGee, 1966) nevertheless,
by some that in one specific type of adjustmental crisis, a
suicidal crisis, untrained persons can be taught specific responses and/or that naive caring is enough, and logic notwith-
standing, "suicide prevention" programs, soliciting suicidal
calls and deploying benevolent lay people to intercept them by
phone, have sprung up with accelerating frequency over the past
decade and a half, inspired chiefly by the establishment of the
Los Angeles Suicide Prevention Center (LASPC) (Helig, 1968) in
1958. This pioneer center, of course, was founded by the NIMH
as a support facility for the ground-breaking research efforts
of psychologists Norman Farberow and Edwin Shneidman in the
previously tabooed area of suicidal behavior. Subsequently, the
LASPC staff began cautiously to experiment with the use of volunteer non-professionals to relieve the staff of some of their
burgeoning clinical responsibilities and to facilitate research,
and this feature of the program caught the public fancy. A
grass-roots "suicide prevention" movement, in effect, resulted,
sweeping the country with near-evangelical fervor and little
rational restraint. It unfortunately has not been clearly recognized that the typical autonomous, lay-operated "suicide prevention" service bears little resemblance to the original LASPC
model. The non-professional staff at the LASPC, in the first
place, execute a restricted function (answering phone calls during the day) under the watchful eye and continuing supervision
of the professional staff while a cadre of graduate students

handle the so-called "Night Watch" by themselves. The total LASPC operation also is a highly professional and primarily re-search-oriented "suicide prevention" program which has little in common with the typical free-standing, lay-operated answer-ing and referral service that has adopted the same generic name.

The contagion of the lay "suicide prevention" movement--however illogical or insubstantial its theoretical base--demands careful, critical analysis of the phenomenon.

It may be noted, first, that a recent survey (McGee, 1966) of 40 such programs across the country (about a 75% sample) re-veals that only 31% in actuality operate with a wholly non-pro-fessional staff and that over two-thirds of the programs are or have become in part or entirely professional in composition, providing indirect confirmation of the proposition that the basic concept of a non-professional emergency service of this or any other type is not viable. Concomitantly, another de-tailed appraisal of a smaller sample of ten representative "sui-cide prevention" programs (Whittemore, 1970) reveals the same trend toward professionalization and a related change in the direction of broadening of the scope of these programs from the original, narrow "suicide prevention" base to encompass "crisis intervention" in general. Most of these programs have, for one thing, either expanded their original "suicide prevention" titles to include "crisis intervention" or have given up the narrower "suicide prevention" appellation entirely in favor of a "crisis intervention" designation. Concomitantly, utilization statistics for the sampled programs demonstrate that less than 10% of the calls to these ostensible "suicide prevention" cen-ters involve suicidal attempts and only one-fourth involve either attempts or threats. Three-fourths of the calls, *i.e.*, to the typical "suicide prevention" center are non-suicidal in nature! (Nearly 40% of the less than 10% of the calls repre-senting actual attempts, furthermore, are placed by third parties who happen to be on or to come on the scene, rather than by the person attempting suicide.) Recent data from the LASPC (Shneidman and Mandelkorn, 1970) demonstrate the same par-adox more emphatically: less than 2% of the calls to this proto-typical "suicide prevention" center involve actual attempts and only 10% involve either attempts or impulses. This ubiquitous finding puts in clear question the theoretical rationale for "suicide prevention" as a unique type of clinical operation, identifiably different from "crisis intervention" in general and correlatively, supports the argument that there is a pre-eminent need for wide-ranging professional skills in emergency mental health programs of this nature.

Another line of evidence challenging the rationale for nar-rowly-conceived, lay-operated "suicide prevention" programs is

that emerging from research on the apparent antithesis between
the suicide-attempter and the suicide-completer--or the "unsuccessful" and the "successful" suicide, to put it in paradoxical
terms. A number of studies describe (McGee, 1966; Beall, 1969;
Shneidman and Farberow, 1970) the typical attempter as a woman,
who tends in personality pattern to be a dependent/hysteric, pro-
testing against the actual or threatened loss of or rejection
by a "significant other," and employing a non-lethal method of
attempting suicide. The typical completer, by contrast, is a
man, who manifests independence in interpersonal relations and
underlying feelings of alienation, and who employs a lethal
method of self-destruction. It has been remarked (Fulton-DeKalb
Emergency Mental Health Service, 1967) that the act of suicide,
for the completer, represents an "assertive" rather than a de-
featist action--an active, ideological commitment to death, while
the attempter's suicidal gesture by contrast represents an atten-
tion-getting "cry for help," to borrow Farberow and Shneidman's
(1961) poetic phrase--a desperate but paradoxically self-abort-
ing effort to escape life-stress while clinging to life. It
follows, as several recent studies (Fulton-DeKalb Emergency
Mental Health Service, 1967; Seiden, 1971) have demonstrated,
that it is the attempter, not the completer, who is attuned to
and responds to the naive, outreaching efforts of a "suicide prevention" service while, ironically, the completer, the putative
target of such a service, is unaffected. This finding puts in
serious question the whole rationale for "suicide prevention"
programs, conceived of as rescue services, as indicated.

A further consideration is that the necessarily circumscribed and naive helping efforts of the lay "suicide prevention"
worker, which have become somewhat ritualized (Farberow, Helig &
Litman, 1970; NIMH Center for Studies of Suicide Prevention, undated) and which ordinarily involve first an attempt to gauge
the "lethality" of suicidal intent by direct questioning, and
then a summons to police or ambulance or a referral to a mental
health professional, may not only not be helpful but may aggra-
vate problems. With the genuinely suicidal, potential completer, for example, crude "helping" efforts of this type may repel
and totally alienate the already estranged completer and firm
his covert rejection of others and suicidal resolve. Thomas
Szasz, among others, (Macks, 1971; Szasz, 1971) lately has pro-
tested against the so-called "coercive" intervention of zealous
non-professional "suicide prevention" workers and has questioned
the ethics and propriety of involuntary rescue or pressurized referral. The lay suicide worker's blunt interrogation of callers
to determine the "lethality" of their suicidal intentions appears also suspect. Such questioning may, as indicated, repel
the sensitive, already-alienated, potential completer; it may
also have a dangerous power of suggestion for the hysteric
attempter. The very act of labelling and promoting a "suicide

prevention" service, in fact, may suggest suicidal ideation to this type of personality and thus paradoxically introduce a suicide risk. (Callers have been known (McGee, 1966) to manufacture suicidal ideation in order to justify use of such a service.) At the same time, there is evidence that "lethality" ratings by untrained workers have no predictive power and therefore no utility, for they have been found to vary directly with and to reflect the degree of inexperience and level of anxiety of the lay worker rather than the gravity of the suicidal crisis. It has been demonstrated, (Shneidman, 1971) conversely, that "lethality" can be assessed with a very high degree of precision by an experienced psychologist, and the unarguable conclusion is that a delicate clinical judgment is involved for which professional competence is a requisite. There appears, *ergo*, to be no shortcut to nor substitute for professional competence in emergency mental health operations of this type.

It may also be noted that several studies reveal that many or most of the consumers of non-professional "suicide prevention" services have previously had or are currently receiving some type of professional help, which is consistent with the hypothesis that the typical consumer of this type of service is a dependent/hysteric suicide-attempter rather than a completer. This finding suggests that the practice of referring (these already psychiatrically or psychologically sophisticated) callers for professional help is redundant, and the concomitant finding (Whittemore, 1970; Murphy, Wetzel, Swallow & McClure, 1968) that follow-through on such referrals is typically limited supports this judgment. Since referral or rescue are the non-professional suicide worker's chief functions, it would appear that little is actually accomplished by their efforts.

Apart from consideration of the theoretical and clinical implications and consequences of lay-operated "suicide prevention" services, there is, of course, a pragmatic question of economy. The appeal of the program manned by volunteer nonprofessionals lies of course, at base, in the low cost--on paper-- of the service. There are high, indirect costs of utilizing untrained volunteers, however, to substitute for or supplement professionals in the delivery of emergency services of this type--the professionals who organize or provide consultation to the program in the long run spend as much or more time in recruiting, selecting, training, and supervision of the non-professionals as they would in providing direct services and there is simply an indirect rather than a direct expenditure of professional time and skill. There also is, typically, an indirect cost in the form of loss of morale among non-professional workers in this type of program, over a period of time, which compounds the problems of recruitment, training, and supervision. This is reflected in the universally high turnover and

attrition rate among voluntary non-professionals in these programs. The absence of compensation inevitably saps the morale
of volunteer non-professionals and gives rise to some feeling
of exploitation (particularly when there are compensated and un-
compensated staff), and there is also a subtle threat to morale
involved in the covert role conflict that is typically induced
in the fledgling, non-professional mental health worker in the
course of his brief training and abrupt exposure to acute adjustmental problems and crisis situations in the lives of others.
As he gains experience, however superficial, a sense of professional pride and ambition is prematurely awakened and he comes
to think of himself as a member of a professional service and
yet he attains no licit professional status. At the least, sup-
pressed frustration and envy of legitimate (and adequately compensated) professionals are felt, while ultimately many dedi-
cated lay workers abandon their anomalous roles because of the
built-in role conflict--the position of the unpaid non-professional in a "suicide prevention" or other type of emergency
mental health service becomes, in time, psychologically unten-
able.

A parenthetical observation from the LASPC experience and
two other experimental projects (Rioch, Elkers & Flint, undated;
McGee, 1966) in non-degree training of ancillary mental health
personnel is that a minimum of two years of study and training
(involving both course work and field training) has been found
necessary. Since trainees are typically college-educated (or
better) and the training is therefore at a graduate level, a
master's degree in psychology or social work could be earned in
the same time or less, and the conclusion appears to be that
there is no shortcut to professional competence.

The array of theoretical, clinical, and economic arguments
against the use of non-professionals in "suicide prevention"
programs appears to mandate rejection of "crisis intervention"
models of this type and choice of a professionally-staffed
model.

PROFESSIONAL "CRISIS" INTERVENTION" PROGRAMS

Suicide Counseling Associations

Turning, then, to consideration of professionally-staffed
"crisis intervention" programs, at the opposite pole of the pro-
fessional/lay descriptive dimension, there are voluntary associations of professionals for suicide counseling which have emerged
spontaneously, in this country and abroad, at intervals over the

past half-century (Farberow and Shneidman, 1961). These are at base social welfare programs with a religious flavor, usually sponsored by social agencies or church-related organizations. They frequently include mental health paraprofessionals (ministers, physicians, nurses, lawyers, and educators) along with social workers, psychologists, and psychiatrists as mental health professionals; there sometimes is a nucleus of paid professionals as a regular staff. Short-term, emergency counseling is offered either indirectly (by phone) or directly (in person) in identified suicidal crises. These programs are narrow in compass, by definition, and are limited in an operational sense by their voluntary and loosely-organized character. The use of volunteer professionals represents of course a significant paper economy, but entails a devitalizing sacrifice of efficiency and control. Attrition among the volunteer professionals is high, and the viability of programs of this ilk is a direct function of the degree of dedication and emotional stamina of their leadership. Typically, there is a low survival rate.

Emergency Psychiatric Services

A different "crisis intervention" model utilizes professionals on a compensated basis, providing for better-coordinated services and more sustained participation. One variant of the compensated professional model is the "emergency psychiatric services" type of program (NIMH, undated; Lamb, Heath and Downing, 1969; Weiss, Straight, Houts and Voten, 1969; Furman, undated). These services typically are linked to a hospital emergency room and patterned after E. R. services. The staff ordinarily consists of psychiatric residents, who provide brief diagnostic screening for hospital admission or stopgap chemotherapy to E. R. "walk-ins" or via home visitations. The model is operationally narrow and limited in its conceptualization of "crisis intervention" in terms of occasional, (rudimentary,) medically-oriented surveillance rather than more comprehensive, continued psychotherapeutic management. Programs of this type have been inspired (in the financial as well as ideological sense) chiefly by the Community Mental Health Services Act of 1963, which stipulated that emergency mental health services must be provided in order for any facility to qualify for federal funds as a community mental health center, and they have proliferated in the past decade as a kind of band-wagon phenomenon with little conceptual programming.

"Crisis Counseling" Programs

An alternative model involving compensated professionals is what may be termed a "crisis counseling" model. In contrast to the "emergency psychiatric services" type of program, this is a conceptually more comprehensive, psychotherapeutically oriented rather than medically/diagnostically oriented model, with a focus on indirect, phone intervention rather than direct, face-to-face contact and at the same time on more in-depth response to a wide range of crisis situations. There are few examples reported of this progressive model, but, as previously intimated, many "suicide prevention" programs appear to be evolving into a broader, more professional "crisis intervention" format and hence to be converging on the "crisis counseling" model.

None of the reported "crisis counseling" services, however, satisfies a criterion of operational comprehensiveness, although there is conceptual breadth, because they are limited to telephone counseling and do not provide follow-up care. Invariably they depend upon referral to other professionals or mental health services for further or continued psychotherapeutic help. In one or two programs, provision for continued psychological care is made in indirect fashion, by housing separate "crisis intervention" and regular outpatient services under the same programmatic roof, so that "crisis" cases can be followed at least within the same facility if not by the same professional (*cf.* the program of the Massachusetts Mental Health Center) (NIMH, undated)), but there is still in such instances a clinically inefficient break in the continuity of care, and an artificial conceptual distinction is drawn between "crisis intervention" and "regular" psychotherapy. Ideally, a fully comprehensive "crisis counseling" model would provide for continuity of care by utilizing the same professional staff for crisis and follow-up counseling and thus would satisfy a threefold criterion of comprehensive, compensated, professional services.

A Comprehensive "Crisis Counseling" Program

One program in Florida emulates such a theoretically ideal, comprehensive, "crisis counseling" model: the Escambia County Community Mental Health Center in Pensacola. From published reports, at least, it appears to be unique in this respect and therefore bears detailed examination and description for heuristic purposes.

At the core of this comprehensive, "crisis counseling" program is a duality of roles assumed by the professional staff

of the outpatient unit of the Center, as a logical consequence
of the fact that emergency mental health services are conceptualized as an integral aspect of or an extension of regular
outpatient services, not as a discontinuous system. In this
program, every staff-member in rotation takes a shift on a
twenty-four-hour emergency or "crisis intervention" schedule
which has been tabbed "Crisis Call." The professional on "Crisis Call" is responsible for managing all calls received during
his shift, whether day or night and whatever the nature of the
call or contact (whether emergency or routine, and whether by
phone or "walk-in"); day or night, the staff-member on "Crisis
Call" executes the same full range of professional functions,
assessing the degree of urgency and the psychological needs in
each case, responding as immediately and actively (in a psychotherapeutic sense) as is required; and offering further counseling or consultation as needed.

     The telephone is the preferred medium for "crisis counsel-
ing" (or"crisis consultation") within this framework, bridging
physical distance and the ritualistic delays of traditional
scheduling-by-appointment, immediately clarifying needs and
coordinating helping efforts in the course of third-party referral or "crisis consultation", and dispelling some of the
stigma and negative mystique of mental health services for the
naive caller. "Walk-in" crisis cases are seen at the Center
during the day, but are not solicited actively, for experience
demonstrates that in this locale at least, the typical "walk-in"
client is *not* in crisis, and is more likely to have stopped by
the Center out of curiosity or on idle impulse, or to have been
arbitrarily remanded to the Center by another social or health
agency, or private professional, in mechanical fashion, for no
clear reason. If a crisis is experienced in a "walk-in" case,
it is frequently experienced by a third party (parent, teacher,
spouse) who conveys the resisting "patient" into the august
presence of the professional for judgment (as "crazy" or "sick")
and "treatment" (perceived as magical exorcism or as restraint,
by confinement or chemical means). Partly for this reason,
counseling and psychotherapy in this program are family- and
relationship- centered, rather than individually focused, and
consultation with allied, "caretaker" agencies and paraprofessionals is emphasized--the program is comprehensive in this
sense as well as in the sense of continuity of care.

     (At night, the telephone is the exclusive medium for "Cris-
is Call" and reliance is placed explicitly and realistically on
indirect, verbal intervention rather than direct confrontation.
If, however, physical intervention in some form is required (in
the event, *e.g.*, of a serious suicidal attempt or a financial
emergency) the "Crisis Call" staff-member calls, of course, on
other emergency resources in the community and can expertly

monitor and coordinate rescue efforts or welfare assistance.)

"Crisis Call" has its own phone number to enhance visibil-
ity of the service in the community and so identify and expedite
crisis calls. All calls are screened through the Center switch-
board and receptionist during daytime office hours and through a
commercial answering service at night and on week-ends. The
staff-member on call, day or night, must remain accessible by
phone at all times; at night, however, he takes calls in his
home, relayed to him by the answering service.

The mode of reimbursement for night "Crisis Call" is via
compensatory time. This means of reimbursement is not only
extraordinarily economical for the Center and community (128
hours a week of professional time on night "Crisis Call," *e.g.*,
costs but 21 hours of compensatory time), but also appears to
have some psychological advantages over monetary compensation
from the staff's point of view. Time off from daily responsibilities is highly valued by professionals, and it appears also
to lend a certain dignity to "overtime" work. From an accounting and administrative point of view, compensation in the form
of time is a more flexible commodity than money and it has the
distinct advantage of being an invisible and readily absorbed
expense, requiring no direct, budgetary defense or justification. This highly effective system of compensation of course is
a mechanical byproduct of the duality of roles assumed by the
outpatient staff in this program.

From an economic, mechanical, and clinical point of view,
the comprehensive "crisis counseling" model appears to function
in a highly efficient manner. (The only drawback, if it be such,
is a subtle one that arises from the overlapping roles played
by the staff; some Center clients perceive the night "Crisis
Call" staff as being "on call" for other staff, in the medical,
group practice tradition, rather than as providing an ancillary,
outreach service, and this results occasionally in abuse of the
service and exploitation of the night staff--in the latter's
opinion. The problem is resolved on an individual basis by the
night "Crisis Call" staff-member, with the caller and/or his
regular therapist, if and when it occurs.)

Preliminary utilization statistics on night "Crisis Call"
tend to confirm this impression. The average frequency of calls
per evening is two (which is consistent with projection from
other "crisis counseling" programs, taking into account a local
population of about 200,000); this rate appears to reflect a sufficient need for and use of the service without overburdening
the night "Crisis Call" staff. Virtually all (90%) of the
night calls are appropriate, in the sense that they are of a
clinical rather than information-giving character and require

half to three-quarters of an hour of intensive phone counseling or consultation, on the average. Furthermore, fully half of the calls are classified as "extremely urgent" and three-quarters are classified as either "moderately""or "extremely urgent". Night "Crisis Call," *ergo*, appears to answer a genuine and unique need, and the impression is that the active and appropriate use, of and positive response to the service by the local community is a direct consequence of its professional character and the feature of continuity of care. It is of interest in this regard, that in over two-thirds of the cases, follow-up counseling is scheduled, while in 20%, a single intensive, phone counseling or consultation session suffices, and only about 12% of the calls entail referral to other emergency health or welfare resources in the community. It may also be noted incidentally, that some callers explicitly respond to and make use of the protective shield of anonymity that can be offered by a phone counseling service, and that some also use night "Crisis Call" on a repeated basis to the exclusion of other, direct modes of psychotherapeutic help--providing testimony for the effectiveness of indirect phone counseling as a unique mode of psychotherapy.

It may further be noted that fewer than half of the night callers (41%) are new to psychotherapeutic help while the majority have had some prior contact with mental health professionals. It could be argued from this that this program largely is tapping a population of already-identified consumers of mental health services and that its value therefore is attenuated. This, however, is a common finding among "crisis intervention" programs of all types, as previously has been suggested, and appears more simply to bear out the axiom that most individuals making an unstable adjustment have a history of unstable adjustment.

The conclusion, from this comparative survey of "crisis intervention" models and detailed examination of the comprehensive "crisis counseling" model, is that the latter model, satisfying as it does the criteria of compensated professionalism and of conceptual and operational comprehensiveness, and featuring indirect, phone counseling as a primary therapeutic modality, approximates an ideal "crisis intervention" type.

NOTE: An altered version of this chapter appears in *Crisis Intervention and Counseling by Telephone*, edited by David Lester and Gene Brockoff, published by Charles C. Thomas, Springfield, 1973.

REFERENCES

Beall, L. The dynamics of suicide, a review of the literature, 1897-1965. *Bulletin of Suicidology*, 1969, 2-16.

Farberow, N. L. and Shneidman, E. S. (Eds.). *The cry for help*. New York: McGraw-Hill, 1961.

Farberow, N. L. and Shneidman, E. S. A survey of agencies for the prevention of suicide. In Farberow, N. L. and Shneidman, E. S. (Eds.). *The cry for help*. New York: McGraw-Hill, 1961.

Farberow, N. L., Helig, S. N., and Litman, R. E. Evaluation and management of suicidal persons. In Shneidman, E. S., Farberow, N. L., and Litman, R. E. (Eds.) *The Psychology of suicide*. New York: Science House, 1970.

Furman, S. S. *Community mental health services in Northern Europe*. Bethesda, NIMH., USPHS. Publication #1407.

Fulton-DeKalb Emergency Mental Health Service: First Annual Report (August, 1966-August, 1967). Atlanta, Fulton & DeKalb Health Depts.

Helig, S. M., Farberow, N. L., Litman, R. E., & Shneidman, E. S. "Non-professional volunteers in a suicide prevention center," In Shneidman, E. S, Farberow, N. L., & Litman, R. E. (Eds.) *The psychology of suicide*. New York: Science House, 1970.

Helig, S. M. The Los Angeles Suicide Prevention Center. In Farberow, N. L. (Ed)., *Proceedings of the Fourth International Conference for Suicide Prevention*, Los Angeles: Delmar, 1968.

Lamb, H. R., Heath, D. & Downing, J. J. (Eds.). *Handbook of Community Mental Health Practice*. San Francisco: Jossey-Bass, 1969.

Macks, V. W. "Suicide prevention-Mental Health 'Oppression'". *Social work*. 1971, January, Pp. 102-104.

McGee, R. K. *Development and organization of suicide prevention centers*. Paper read at First Annual Symposium, Community Mental Health Services, Georgia Mental Health Institute, Atlanta, November, 1966.

McGee, R. K. *Non-professionals as mental health workers in counseling and testing.* Paper read at American Psychological Association, New York, September, 1966.

McGee, R. K. The Manpower problem in suicide prevention. In Farberow, N. L. (Ed.). *Proceedings of the Fourth International Conference for Suicide Prevention.* Los Angeles: Delmar, 1968.

Murphy, E. G., Wetzel, R., Swallow, C., and McClure, J. N., Jr. *Who calls The Suicide Prevention Center, a study of 55 self-callers.* In N. Farberow (Ed.), *Proceedings of the Fourth International Conference for Suicide Prevention.* Los Angeles: Delmar, 1968.

NIMH Center for Studies of Suicide Prevention. *Training record in suicidology.* Chevy Chase.

NIMH Public Information Branch. *Emergency Services.* Washington: U.S. Government Printing Office, U.S.P.H.S. Publication #1477.

Rioch, M. J., Elkers, C., and Flint, A. A. *Pilot project in training mental health counselors.* Washington, U. S. Government Printing Office, U.S.P.H.S. Publication #1254.

Seiden, R. quoted remarks. *Behavior Today,* 1971, March 29, P.3.

Shneidman, E. S. and Farberow, N. L. Attempted and committed suicides. In Shneidman, E. S., Farberow, N. L., and Litman, R. E. (Eds.). *The psychology of suicide.* New York: Science House, 1970.

Shneidman, E. S. and Mandelkorn, P. How to prevent suicide. In E. S. Shneidman, N. L. Farberow, & R. E. Litman (Eds.), *The psychology of suicide.* New York: Science House, 1970.

Shneidman, E. S. Perturbation and lethality as precursors of suicide in a gifted group. *Life-threatening behavior,* 1971, *1,* 23-45.

Szasz, T. The ethics of suicide. *Intellectual Digest,* 1971, Vol. 2, 53-55.

Weisz, A. E., Staight, D. C., Houts, P. S., and Voten, M. P. Suicide threats, suicide attempts, and the emergency psychiatrist. In Farberow, N. L. (Ed.). *Proceedings of the*

Fourth International Conference for Suicide Prevention. Los Angeles, Delmar, 1968.

Whittemore, K. R. *Ten Centers.* Atlanta (privately printed), 1970.

5: THERAPIST DEMANDS

Crisis intervention is a field which has grown rapidly despite the absence of a well articulated, generally accepted model of the crisis worker's role. In the following chapter, Nancy Sebolt presents some of the challenges faced by crisis therapists as they pursue a service role which is explicitly described. The role is promulgated as one of providing rapid help through a relationship in which the client and therapist are equals in negotiating the structure and goals of the intervention. This equality, which Sebolt sees as contrasting with the assymetry of usual therapy situations, requires that seasoned professionals abandon previous biases and non-professionals develop special human skills.

The role which Sebolt favors for the crisis worker is one of great flexibility. Insofar as the client is permitted to reveal his own wants, the worker must be prepared to offer himself to meet immediate needs for warmth, human feeling, and model behavior. Doing so, according to Sebolt, will often involve difficulty and personal threat for the worker. Further, the intimacy level dictated may be particularly difficult to achieve for the professional, if his training has emphasized the maintenance of distance and control in helping relationships. In any event, the crisis worker may face personal anxieties and institutional role conflicts which challenge his functioning. Where these problems act to prevent the crisis worker from utilizing his human strengths in the relationship, Sebolt feels that he becomes less effective in his intervention.

Given the traditional role which Sebolt would have the crisis worker adopt, several questions arise. One issue discussed in the introduction and the McColskey chapter: should professionals or non-professionals be primary workers in crisis centers? Here, Sebolt grants that highly trained personnel offer advantages in their ability to quickly and accurately assess situations. On the other hand, it is the less experienced worker who may be best able to mobilize his human resources on the client's behalf, unencumbered by a sensed conflict with

"medical model" standards of detachment and objectivity. Another
question, less clearly answered by Ms. Sebolt relates to training and selection (see chapters by Bleach, and Berman). Ms.
Sebolt does not make it clear whether the proposed model for
crisis work requires careful screening for people who are apt
to most successfully meet the challenges, or whether the human
skills can be acquired by most people, given adequate training
or supervision. Given that the role of crisis worker is specified as an atraditional, stressful one, these questions of
training and selection might well be asked of professional populations as well as non-professional.

CRISIS INTERVENTION AND ITS DEMANDS

ON THE CRISIS THERAPIST

Nancy Sebolt

Western Missouri Mental Health Center

Kansas City, Missouri

This paper will not try to present background materials, theory, or didactic material on Crisis Intervention. This has been aptly done by Lindemann, (1965), Caplan and Parad (1965), Rapoport (1965, 1962), and others. This is rather an attempt to look at the demands on and the challenges to the therapist-helping person which the Crisis approach elicits. Secondly, the intent is to explore the possibility that these demands and challenges offer some insight into the lack of the wide-spread use of Crisis Intervention techniques.

In the past twenty years, the Mental Health and associated helping professions have flirted with crisis theory. While many programs have adopted this approach to their ongoing services, others, including Community Mental Health Centers, have been reluctant to either adopt or even experiment with it. They persist in maintaining a program that has a repertoire of treatment services into which a client is slotted upon applying to the agency. Unfortunately, if a client does not fit into the existing "treatment repertoire", then he is diagnosed as unmotivated or too disorganized for treatment and is either left to his own change devices or simply placed on medication.

> Traditionally, poor people have been com-
> pelled to adapt their life style to the
> tangled systems of social agencies. Those
> who could not conform to this social sys-
> tem were deprived of services.
> (Pierson, 1970; p. 48)

This lack of acceptance by Mental Health and helping professions of Crisis Intervention seems surprising in light of its
reported effectiveness with lower socioeconomic people (Pierson,
1970; Sunley, 1968; Sager, 1970). Its practical and problem-
oriented approach is more in keeping with the way of life of
these people than the classical psychotherapy approach which
many programs, including Community Mental Centers, cling to so
persistently.

In the May 9, 1969 issue of *Time* Magazine, an article
"Psychiatry's New Approach: Crisis Intervention" spoke of Crisis
Intervention as being heralded as the third revolution in the
mental health field. The first revolution was the discovery
that the insane were neither demons or criminals, and the second, Freud's development into the emotional topography of the
mind. In each revolution we see a step further in the acceptance and the assessment of the person with the emotional problem. The progression has been from the demon or criminal role
to that of patient with its many implications of dependency,
illness, and helplessness to that of a person with a problem
who needs help. Crisis Intervention does not view crisis and
stress as illness but rather as a normative behavior with the
underlying assumption that having problems does not mean that
one is sick.

> The person remains a *person* from the begin-
> ning to the end of the relationship, He
> does not need to become a *patient* for ther-
> apy to work. Indeed, the approach is oriented
> toward preventing the patient syndrome from
> occurring whenever possible.
> (O'Connell, 1970; P. 245)

In the following pages will be discussed some important aspects of doing Crisis Intervention which by its very nature
places pressure and stress on the therapist. Delineated herein
are the factors, indeed the personal cost, which must be taken
into account when one is considering or is actively involved in
Crisis Intervention. These factors may also be the clues to
the reluctance of many professional people to accept or even to
try the crisis approach. While Crisis theory is in keeping with
professional ethics and principles, it also goes against much
of the past and current teachings, particularly in the area of
non-involvement of the therapist.

Immediate Assessment and Help

In doing Crisis Intervention, there is immediate and con-

tinual pressure on the therapist to assess the problem, situation, and person or family and to begin the treatment-helping
process. "One does what one can as rapidly as possible." (Rusk,
p.27). Many times the crisis therapist must begin the inter-
vention-treatment before there is time to obtain much data. The
experienced worker has more of an advantage in Crisis Intervention than the inexperienced worker or student-trainee, having
a backlog of experience, a more integrated picture of individual,
family, and system dynamics, and more self confidence.

The skillfulness required for a quick and accurate assessment is one of the difficulties in teaching Crisis Intervention
to trainees and/or students. On the other hand, the trainee
and student would not have necessarily incorporated the assumption that non-involvement by the therapist-helping person is of
utmost importance to the treatment process. Thus, the trainee
and student often shows less reluctance to permit a desirable
level of emotional involvement with clients than do staff persons.

Examples of intervention before much data can be gathered
are the cases of the very hysterical person, the out-of-control
child who is hurting himself or others, or the very withdrawn
person. In these cases the crisis therapist may need to establish some controls and contact with the person before going any
further in the interview.

> Crisis psychiatry constitutes a rather severe
> test of a therapist's ego strength in that
> multiple systems and variables must be con-
> sidered in a very brief time in order that
> very significant and at times even life and
> death decisions be made. (Rusk, p.26)

Non-traditional Role

The role of the crisis therapist is not a traditional
one. There is some comfort in the traditional role of the therapist-helping person being the one to set the tone of the interview, do the assessment, and then set the goals for treatment.
In Crisis Intervention, the therapist is involved *with* the
client in working on the problem: thus, they become "partners in
the problem-solving process." The message is that they (the
client) and their opinions are important and that you (the crisis therapist) are not there to take over. The goals are set by
mutual agreement between client and therapist. This mutual
agreement reveals the therapist's ability to work with and to
compromise in the setting of goals, demonstrating an attitude

that can be readily identified by the client. Herein is a dras-
tic change from the traditional role of the therapist who often
sets the rules, limits, and goals in the therapy relationship.
It also changes the relationship from an assymetrical one, with
the therapist on a pedestal, to a more reciprocal one.

Active and Involved

The crisis approach puts the crisis therapist in the role
of taking an active, direct, and involved role. In Crisis Intervention, the therapist is expected to show reactions, feelings, and involvement. This means that the therapist is involved and does not merely reflect. The crisis therapist might use
some of his own experiences or might reach out in affection to
someone. Physical touch and reaching out is a technique frequently used in Crisis Intervention. Physical reaching out is
threatening to the therapist who is accustomed to a neutral position where he does not have to show feelings, voice his own
opinions, or show commitment. In Crisis Intervention, the therapist becomes much more of a real person in that he shows by his
reactions and responses what is happening within himself. The
crisis therapist is there to reflect reality, and reality does
not sit passively and mirror feelings back to the client. The
crisis therapist responds as a person giving pertinent feedback to the client as to how he comes across, is perceived, and
is responded to by others.

> To withhold one's self as a person and to deal
> with the other person as an object does not
> have a high probability of being helpful.
> (Rogers, 1958; P.10)

Aggressive Role

The role of the crisis therapist is an active and aggressive
one as he moves in for data, assesses the problem, situation,
and people, presents a picture to the client of what is going
on, and offers ways of dealing with the problem. The therapist's
aggressiveness may range from moving in and setting verbal or
physical limits, or the breaking into the life style of the withdrawn possibly catatonic person, to the use of touching to
soothe a frightened person. The crisis therapist conveys an
important message of being in command of the situation and thus
able to offer direction out of the problem. The extent of command and taking carge by the crisis therapist should be determined by the situation and what is called for in order to help

the client. This is in contrast to classical psychotherapy where the therapist stays neutral.

> Up to the present there has been a wide-
> spread tendency to equate action with
> 'acting out.' In psycho-analysis the
> urge to act has been treated as suspect;
> it has been viewed as emotional and as
> a source of resistance; it can bring de-
> struction. Psychoanalytic process thus
> puts a damper on action.
> (Ackerman, 1967; p.14)

In one particular situation where a fifteen year old girl used sleeping as an escape mechanism and had been asleep for one and a half days, it was necessary to sit on, tickle, slap, and yell at this girl in order to bring her out of her sleep-withdrawal state. It can be assumed that not everyone would feel comfortable in this therapeutic endeavor. In fact, another staff person had to do crisis support with a psychiatric resi-dent who was ready to admit the girl but who became a staunch supporter of Crisis Intervention when he saw the girl able to talk about her concerns and what caused the withdrawal.

Living Example

In crisis theory the therapist is himself a living, breath-ing, and experiencing example. The therapist's own feelings, security, and confidence in handling the problem becomes mag-netic to the troubled person. The therapist's obvious confi-dence in his own capacity to understand and help offers much ego support to the client. In a way, the crisis therapist must have a certain charisma that immediately attracts and catches people. After the attraction, the therapist's skills continue the belief in him that he can help handle the problems.

From the moment that you greet the client until you say 'goodbye,' you should serve as a reflector to the client of what they need to move toward via openness with feelings, ideas, and communication and an ability to arbitrate within a relationship. Merely letting people know what is wrong or how poorly they pre-sent themselves is not helpful unless you can offer both direct-ly through education, insight, and direction or non-directly through example other alternative ways to operate. Unless you are willing to offer alternative ways to functioning, then don't tear down already existing patterns of functioning even if they are destructive. This is predicated upon the assumption that destructive functioning is better than no functioning at all.

Along this line, I personally wonder if this lack of a living, breathing, feeling--a real--person is not the problem of many of the people that I've met who have been in psychotherapy or analysis for years and who operate in a stiff, intellectual way--much like a thinking zombie with no feelings.

If there is a co-therapist in a crisis session or crisis group, then your relationship, that is how you communicate, handle disagreements, react and respond to one another, is living proof of the goals toward which you will try to encourage the client to move. Teaching, role playing, or any other technique is really no substitute for the liveliness of the therapist's own humanity in communicating. By being real there is exhibited a living example of communication.

Elicits Strong Feelings

The crisis approach elicits strong feelings of the client towards the crisis therapist. At times these feelings will range from close, warm feelings demonstrated by a hug or a kiss to anger, particularly if the therapist has to set some limits. The therapist's active involvement, obvious respect for the client, and the showing of feelings often produce a rapid and intense trusting, dependent transference. It is this omnipotent transference figure which the crisis therapist utilizes to cut into the maladaptive patterns, to allow ventilation of feelings, and to offer alternative ways of operating.

For example, I have been in interviews or groups where other staff people have become quite "uptight" when a client has reached out to embrace or to kiss me in appreciation for the help given to them. What a surprise it must be to the client if a therapist-helping person is uncomfortable and unable to accept the real expression of warm feelings.

Variety in Depth and Length of Involvement

The length of and the depth of the involvement with a client varies greatly and depends on the client, his needs, and his situation. With people who have many inner, family, and community resources to fall back upon, it may call for only one or two interviews and then the client handles things on his own. In almost all cases, we should respect the client's wish to try things on his own. It is a rule of thumb in Crisis Intervention that the client's wish to try things on his own is respected. To do otherwise would be to move the relationship toward the

more classical psychotherapeutic model or to foster greater dependency upon the therapist. The exception to this would be a
life or death situation with either a suicidal or homicidal person. Insistance that change and healthy behavior can only be
obtained at a mental health agency or with professional people
is both absurd and contradictory to the crisis message. There
is simply too much evidence that non-professional people in the
community have rendered help to those in stress. Taxicab driv-
ers, hair dressers and barbers, bartenders, in addition to
clergymen or physicians are just some of the cadre of people who
offer advice and assistance to those who are hurting.

In other instances, it may be necessary to become very involved and over an extended period of time.

> One begins where the patient is in regard to
> his ego capacity. Crisis Intervention is no
> place for passive permissiveness. A human
> encounter is called for. One cannot afford
> the luxury of scientific appropriate distance;
> nor is the patient's ego often healthy enough
> for an independent, introspective growth ex-
> perience.   (Rusk, P. 14)

From this perspective, the crisis therapist should supply
whatever nurturing is needed in order to pull things together
for the client. Interestingly enough the popular phrase "getting it together" is precisely the crux of not only psychotherapy but of Crisis Intervention. The aim is the integration of
life experiences. The major difference is that Crisis Intervention is "here and now" life experiences while traditional
therapy deals with past as well as present living, though some
reports would show a concentration on past events. In Crisis
Intervention, the therapist lends help and proceeds with the
expectation that growth can restore functioning to at least the
best previous adaptive level and that the need of therapeutic
involvement will diminish. "Do for others that which they cannot do for themselves, and no more." (Rusk, p. 6) The crisis
therapist must be able to gain satisfaction from helping others
not to be too dependent on him and to be able to make use of
other community resources, thus to be able to "let go."

Flexibility

The demand for flexibility can be both threatening and ex-
hausting to the crisis therapist. First, he must be ready to
respond at any time to a crisis situation, and this means the
juggling of appointments and the moving into and out of things

quickly and with little preparation.

Because people's needs vary and because different things work with different people, the crisis therapist must be well versed in many different approaches. The shifting of emotional gears and the ability to pick up the pace of the client is a needed quality which becomes a high priority due to the rapidity of events. The approach, methods, and techniques will come from the client, his needs, and his interaction with the therapist-helping person. At the Western Missouri Mental Health Center we have found that certain therapists develop skills in a particular area such as working with situations involving death, terminal illness, or drugs. The rest of the team then uses the expertise of this person for consultation, training, or might even float the expert into the interview with them. If the problem situation is known before the interview, then both the "expert" and another staff do the interview. So far we have found no particular problem with the floating in of another staff person providing there is no time lag and both staff persons are comfortable with the introjection of the area expert. Frequently the expert is briefed on the clients situation right in the interview, thus the client is able to observe the communication process between the staff.

Anxiety Provoking

Because of its very intense nature and its emotional demands on the therapist, the crisis approach can be anxiety provoking to the therapist. The crisis therapist is continually called on to deal with people who are experiencing extreme anxiety prompted by emotion laden situations such as death, terminal illness, child abuse, drugs, suicide, etc. which can also promote anxiety in the therapist. It thus becomes expedient that the crisis therapist find some way of dealing with his anxiety regarding the client, the situation, his own efforts, and the outcome. A steady diet of crisis cases with no outlet for affectively dealing with such feelings often results in a crisis therapist himself being in crisis. It should be noted that probably not all professionals will be able to do crisis work or at least not on a steady basis.

A crisis team seems the best way of handling the feelings of the crisis therapists. The team is a group of people in close physical proximity to each other who are comfortable enough with one another to share feelings, able to confront each other, and able to give support to one another. This does not necessarily mean that they work together on specific cases, but that they have access to and can use each other for ventilalation, thinking through, and support.

It is essential that there be some built-in mechanism for the crisis therapists to handle their own feelings and that this be something other than supervision with its many implications of authority, teacher-learner, boss-employee, and other frequently negative connotations. I, as a supervisor and administrator, use the group mechanism for the handling of my feelings after doing a crisis interview.

Unpopular

Lastly, the crisis client-oriented therapist is frequently not popular within the agency or with administration. Tensions can grow within the institution if the therapist becomes an advocate of some of his clients' needs and voices some of the agency's short-comings to the extent that he even suggests changes in the agency program or 'treatment repertoire' so that the agency program is more in keeping with client needs as versus staff needs.

> Sensitivity to the client may often be
> disadvantageous for the organization man.
> If, when confronted with an irregular
> case he rigidly sticks to the organiza-
> tion norms, he usually fares better than
> if he tried to bend the norms of the
> organization to the client's needs or
> if he bothers his superiors with the case.
> Furthermore, contacts with clients is
> usually relatively concentrated on the
> lower levels of the organization; those
> who are successful in their relations with
> clients may find it more difficult to at-
> tain promotion than those who prepare
> themselves for the next, less client
> oriented stages by being more organiza-
> tion than client minded. To sum up:
> to be overly client oriented and to
> transmit client's demands upward is a
> relatively unrewarding experience in
> many organizations. (Etizionia, 1964; P. 100)

Frequently after years of operation or with exceptionally large agencies, the treatment program is more reflective of staff needs than client needs, i.e., agency hours, waiting lists, forms of therapy. This seems particularly applicable in agencies where there is a large training program. Educational and training programs at times are even more behind than agencies in being applicable to client and community needs.

It is necessary to have some administrative support in order to have a crisis program, but even this does not preclude other staff from becoming quite upset over such a program and its effect on other agency services. For example, at my own agency, a community mental health center, we had the backing and support of the superintendent; however, the crisis approach in Children's Intake had impact on the rest of children's services and we had many complaints and negative feelings regarding the lack of inpatient admissions and letting clients go who would make good training cases. The classical child guidance evaluation model of mental status, psychologicals, and social study on every child assures good training material both for evaluations and for treatment, but unfortunately, this does not necessarily serve the best interests, needs, and time of the client.

SUMMARY

Mental health and the helping sciences have come a long way in their short period of existence. The person with emotional problems has come from being seen as possessed by a demon or criminally insane to being viewed as a person who is sick and must assume a patient role in order to obtain help to now being regarded as a person who is experiencing problems in coping with his situation. The outcome for the person with emotional problems has travelled from no hope to possible cure with long term treatment to an expectation of quick return to previous levels of adaptation if help is appropriately given at the right time and suitably focused.

Crisis intervention has brought a whole new dimension to the helping relationship and one that has been lacking: that of the personhood of the therapist-helping person as a living, breathing, and experiencing person. Too long professionals have hidden behind the professional mask of non-involvement.

> One of the important reasons for the professionalization of every field is that it helps to keep distance. In the clinical areas we develop elaborate diagnostic formulations, seeing the person as an object.   (Rogers, 1958; P. 12)

Now the client is seen as a person, not a patient, and evaluated in terms of strength rather than illness. The therapist reacts as a "real" person rather than an intellectual being that reflects

and interjects. The most important aspect of the crisis
approach is the blossoming of the therapist-helping person into
a warm, experiencing being that both reaches out to and responds
to the client's reaching out and responses.

> This is the work of the crisis, the work of
> the therapy to transform ourselves with the
> others, and in this sounding out, to meet
> him and know him.   (O'Connell, 1970, P. 247)

In order to be effective in crisis work, it is my opinion that
the therapist must take all the authority vested by the agency
and use it, and must push from within and without for agency
change.

It is this sincere and caring attitude that has carried
many unexperienced but well meaning helping persons through an
interview or situation with good results. All of our well
thought out and well said statements, directions, and interpretations can go for naught if our actions do not match our words.

I challenge those who would help to become involved and to
risk themselves in relationships with their clients.

REFERENCES

Ackerman, N. W. The future of family psychotherapy, *Expanding theory and practice in family therapy*. New York: Family Service Association of America, 1967.

Caplan, G. & Parad, H. J. A framework for studying families in crisis. In H. J. Parad (Ed.), *Crisis intervention: Selected readings*. New York: Family Service Association of America, 1965.

Etizionia, A. *Modern organizations*. Foundations of Modern Sociology Series. New Jersey: Prentice-Hall, Inc., 1964.

Glad, D. D. & Barnes, R. H. The network of psychiatric services. Paper presented at a symposium on Group Approaches in Programs for Socially Deprived Populations at the Twenty-Seventh Annual Conference on American Group Psychotherapy. San Francisco, California, January, 1965.

Hill, R. Generic features of families under stress. In H. J. Parad (Ed.), *Crisis intervention: Selected readings*. New York: Family Service Association of America, 1965.

Lindemann, E. Symptomalogy and Management of acute grief. In H. J. Parad (Ed.), *Crisis intervention: Selected readings*. New York: Family Service Association of America, 1965.

O'Connell, V. F. Crisis psychotherapy: Person, dialogue, and the organismic event. In J. Fagen and I. L. Shepherd (Eds.), *Gestalt therapy now*. New York: Harper Colophon Books, 1970.

Pierson, A. Social work techniques with the poor. *Social Casework*. Vol. 15, No. 4, October, 1970.

Rapoport, L. The state of crisis: Some theoretical considerations. In H. J. Parad (Ed.), *Crisis intervention: Selected readings*. New York: Family Service Association of America, 1965.

Rogers, C. The characteristics of a helping relationship. *Personnel and Guidance Journal, 37, 1,* July, 1962.

Rusk, T. N. Opportunities in crisis theory. Unpublished paper.

Sager, C. J., Thomas, L., Brayber, M. D., and Waxenberg, B. R. *Black ghetto family in therapy: A laboratory experience*. New York: Grove Press, 1970.

Sunley, R.   New dimensions in reaching out casework.   *Social Work*.   Vol. 13, No. 2, April, 1968.

6: OPERATION OF A CRISIS INTERVENTION CENTER

In many communities, non-professionals manage and staff walk-in or telephone crisis intervention services. In this chapter, Sam Stern describes the development and operation of the Tuscaloosa Crisis Center with an emphasis on procedures and operating policy. This center typifies the organized crisis center operating under the influence of a university based psychology department.

The description highlights the benefits of coordinating crisis services with local agencies already working with the target population, *e.g.*, the police, community mental health center, and courts. The center's policies seem designed to protect the non-professional group from criticism by mental health establishment forces, by retaining the ultimate responsibility in this center with professionals. Other crisis centers operate in a more free wheeling anti-establishment manner rejecting mental health professionals and excluding liaisons with traditional mental health administrators.

The data on the calls received by the center are representative of crisis center experiences and provides an indication of the nature of the population utilizing the service. A comparison of the kind of problems reported by crisis centers with those reported by mental health agencies might suggest modifications of both services to improve matching of the mode of service delivery to the type of crisis (see chapter by Korner).

The Tuscaloosa center has experienced difficulty recruiting Blacks for their staff and has noted little use of the service by Blacks. This raises important questions about designing paraprofessional mental health service for Black communities. Crisis intervention centers seem to be typically utilized by white, young, middle class people who have easy access to telephones and to words as a means toward a solution of their problems.

The difficulties attending the implementation of follow-up procedures noted in this chapter demonstrate how volunteers exert considerable influence over the operation of the center. While follow-up procedures may reduce the effectiveness of hotline services, it seems likely that the surfacing of this reason serves partially as a rationalization to conceal the individual worker's reluctance to be examined. Further discussion of this problem can be found in the chapter by Bleach.

Comparison of the training procedures outlined for the Tuscaloosa center with those proposed in the chapter by Berman, suggests that administrative and supervisory requirements may produce an emphasis on structure rather than on creativity. The description in this chapter does provide an example of a typical organization limited in its scope and capabilities by the constraints arising out of a need for order and control.

In judging the strengths and weaknesses of the Tuscaloosa center, appreciation of the forces which determine the form and nature of this center should enhance planning and development of new services in similar circumstances.

THE TUSCALOOSA COMMUNITY CRISIS INTERVENTION CENTER

Sam Stern

University of Alabama

Tuscaloosa Crisis Center

HISTORY

The Fall of 1970 saw the emergence of a means for dealing with a critical need in Tuscaloosa, a university town of about 60,000 in west, central Alabama. A drug-oriented "hippy" subculture in Tuscaloosa found itself increasingly plagued with problems of drug overdosage, "bad trips" or "bummers", and related phenomena. Individuals with these problems had few, if any, places to turn for help. Many of these persons (sometimes unjustifiably, but sometimes justifiably) dreaded a possible confrontation with law-enforcement authorities in and around Tuscaloosa and they consequently avoided conventional sources of help such as the local hospital, Psychological Clinic, or the University of Alabama Student Health Service. Moreover, some of the drug users harbored a deep resentment and distrust of the "Establishment and its alleged prejudice against and insensitivity to the attitudes of the hippy community.

While the initial impetus for a crisis center were drug-related problems, the crisis center ultimately established was and still is an *all-purpose* center and is not now primarily drug-oriented.

The need for a crisis center was publically advocated by Michael Hughes, a staff member of a Tuscaloosa underground newspaper. However, Hughes was unable to implement his plans. Fortunately, Terry Thomason, a friend of Hughes, did have the time and interest in starting such a center. Hughes informed Thomason that Dr. Michael Dinoff, Director of the Psychological Clinic at the University of Alabama, might be helpful in organizing and staffing the crisis center. Dr. Dinoff soon won the confidence and trust of the drug community. Thomason, Dinoff, Jerry Lowe and Valodi Foster of the Tuscaloosa community, psychology and social work department faculty and graduate students, physicians, lawyers, and clergymen made up the core of the new service organization. Since its inception, numerous other professionals, students, and community people, have played vital roles in keeping the Tuscaloosa Community Crisis Intervention (CC) alive and operating.

During its approximately half-year "gestation", the CC evolved from a drug-oriented focus to a flexible telephone (and, recently, walk-in) service which would offer assistance in all types of crises, called or presented in person involving University students and residents of the Tuscaloosa community.

As a result of initial planning, the law enforcement agencies and courts in and around Tuscaloosa agreed not to wire tap, electronically "bug" or interfere with the CC's operation. Indeed, future events helped to form and cement a friendly and cooperative relationship with the police, a relationship which began to alter pre-existing, stereotyped views that the police were out to arrest every "drug-crazed" hippy in Tuscaloosa.

Much hard work went into creating this cooperative atmosphere. Numerous meetings with police, discussions, verbal commitments and letters of intent had to be arranged. The CC owes much to the helpful, enlightened, trusting laissez-faire attitude which the local law enforcement agencies and courts have generally assumed.

As a result of a vigorous flurry of activity which included cooperation between often antagonistic groups, the intensive training of trainers and volunteers, several mass group meetings, moving into and preparing a building and telephones, the Tuscaloosa Community Crisis Intervention Center was born on December 11, 1970.

PURPOSE OF THE CRISIS CENTER

The purpose of the CC, as expressed in its title, is to provide the caller (C) with at least temporary relief and help during a troublesome or crisis situation. The kind of help offered is typically of a *short-term* variety. That is, the CC does not offer psychotherapy. Interactions are, hopefully, *therapeutic*, though not as a result of psychotherapy *qua* psychotherapy. Our volunteers (Vs) are trained to focus more on the immediate reason for the call (*i.e.*, the caller's distress rather than its long-term causes). The CC V is trained to ascertain whether the circumstances and stresses which prompted the call in the first place are relatively acute or chronic. Though the support and sympathy conveyed may be similar in both cases, supplementary aid might be appropriate for chronic problems, in which case the V would refer the caller to sources of specific and longer term assistance.

STRUCTURE AND OPERATION OF THE CRISIS CENTER

The CC operates 24 hours a day, seven days a week all year. Telephone service consists of 4 lines, the fourth line used primarily for outgoing calls to the professional backup and personal incoming calls. The three lines sequentially ring to the same dialed number. A separate phone, in cooperation with Alcoholics Anonymous, enables alcoholics or their family members to obtain help from members of AA via the CC.

There are five levels of workers in the CC: the Vs (Volunteer), professional backups, trainer-volunteer group (the so-called "Thursday Meeting"), Executive Director and the Board of Directors.

Our front line service workers are telephone Vs. These are trained Vs who answer the phones and are continually involved in crisis intervention. To work on a telephone Vs must be at least 18 years old; Vs under 18 are assigned to secretarial and sometimes (depending on qualifications) scheduling duty. They are permitted to answer the phones only after they complete the training program and turn 18 years of age. Vs work a four hour shift which is arranged on a "sign-up sheet" in the phone room. Because of manpower shortages, some Vs chose to work two or more 4-hour shifts. Consecutive 4-hour shifts, however, are discouraged since extended phone duty is believed to lower one's effective coping with crisis situations. Despite this, during a few periods of critical Vs shortage, some individuals worked up to 12 consecutive hours. We try to keep such marathon vigils to an absolute minimum.

Seven CC members voluntarily are responsible for scheduling the 6 shifts on their chosen day. They ensure that someone is on duty at all times. This sometimes means that they themselves must fill in any vacancies they cannot fill, or if someone does not show up for their shift and cannot be located.

Moreover, Vs usually work in pairs, preferably one male and one female, since some callers insist on speaking to a V of his or her own sex, or to someone of the opposite sex. While one V talks on the phone, the other may help locate referral sources in the phone room, call a backup professional if necessary, or

handle additional incoming calls. During V shortages, some individuals have had to work alone. When several phone calls came
in simultaneously or before a previous call was completed, the
V was forced to take the most important call and request that
the less distressed call back later.

At the present time, there are approximately 100 Vs of whom
50 to 60 work at least one shift a week. The male:female ratio
is approximately even though females sometimes outnumber males.
Most of our Vs are students at the University of Alabama though
an increasingly large proportion are residents of Tuscaloosa
such as housewives and businessmen. Toward improving the CC's
community-contacts,non-student Vs are needed and encouraged.

The training program at the CC consists of groups of 10-15
people with two co-leaders. These trainers are experienced
workers and typically graduate level students in the helping professions. The groups meet once or twice weekly usually for 2-3
hours each session. Training lasts about one month (meeting
twice weekly) or two months (once weekly) for approximately
24-30 hours of actual, intensive training. Recently, the CC successfully experimented with a marathon training session which
accomplished most of the required training in the span of one
weekend. Starting with the marathon group, we administered the
MMPI to the trainers and Vs with the ultimate goal of being able
to predict successful Vs based on MMPI profiles. We are continuing this research with subsequent groups. After the completion
of formal training, the group continues to meet less frequently
to discuss problems and to keep abreast of the latest CC developments.

The training program consists of several phases: 1) reading, discussion and critique the CC training manual (which contains basic information and procedures), 2) sensitivity training techniques for enhancement of group cohesiveness, 3) role
playing procedures using special "Teletrainer" training telephones loaned from South Central Bell Telephone, 4) observation
of experienced Vs taking crisis calls, and 5) supervised crisis
intervention including the intermittant monitoring and crit-
iquing of calls.

The training telephones add a great deal of realism and
some appropriate tension to the role playing. Typically, one
person volunteers to "call in" with a crisis he makes up or is
suggested by the trainer while another volunteers to accept the
call. If no one volunteers, "Vs" are randomly selected from
name cards. After the role play is completed, the interaction
is discussed and critiqued with the group and role players.
Strengths and weaknesses are pointed out in a constructive manner.

Also, trainees receive practice in entering the role played into a practice logbook. This entry is also critiqued.

The training procedure serves as a screening device as well, and a minority of the trainees do not make it through the training period. The majority of these drop out on their own accord. A few are 'passed' on a borderline basis and are subsequently closely monitored. A few others are asked outright to leave, perhaps with encouragement to try again in the future in a different training group. The trainers are requested to screen out those individuals whom they feel are overly rigid, prejudiced, moralizers, emotionally unstable or considered ineffective crisis intervenors. We maintain that all Vs are entitled to their own personal beliefs, but that they should keep them to themselves. Moralizing or giving direct advice to a caller is usually vigorously discouraged. Rather, the trainee learns to discuss both sides of an issue or problem, offers various *alternatives* to a problem, but leaves the final decision up to the caller. As with most other rules, there are exceptions to this one, as in the case of life or death suicide or similar situations where immediate, direct advice may be necessary to save a life.

Trainers themselves are screened and selected by other trainers on a "trainer screening committee" subject to final approval by the Board of Directors. Trainees are provided with a separate manual which was compiled by Hermann Witte, a CC V.

All Vs must enter all calls into a logbook, recording the number of each call, the time it came in, the time it ended, the nature of the caller's problem, the resolution (if any) of the problem, and comments. In accordance with our policy of strict anonymity and confidentiality, no identifying information is entered into the logbook, *i.e.*, no names, addresses, phone numbers. Again, in exceptional life or death cases where a name, address and phone number are essential, for example, to rush medical aid to the caller, such information is written on a separate piece of paper and clipped in the logbook. When the crisis is resolved, the paper is destroyed. The CC training manual offers suggestions on how to terminate excessively long calls that are getting nowhere, as well as techniques to draw out inhibited or silent callers who would otherwise make for an unnecessarily brief call. Several bulletin boards in our phone room keep all Vs posted on the latest calls which require longer-term attention.

While our telephone number (205-758-3331) is publicly announced, the CC's location is not. However, it is spread by word of mouth. This avoids a surge of curiosity seekers, yet at the same time allows those persons with problems to actually

come to the CC and receive help in person. These "walk-ins" are
helped in a separate livingroom and not in the phone room.

The CC's next line of workers are the professional backups.
These are professionals such as psychologists, nurses and social
workers who are on call at their work or homes for a 24-hour
period. The backup offers advice and suggestions on any matter
that a V feels unsure about. The backups are especially well
versed in CC policies, and are responsible for decisions which
may have serious legal repercussions.

Ongoing organizational policies are made by the trainer-
volunteer group or "Thursday Group (Meeting)". This group is
comprised of professional backups and Board of Director members
as well as trainers and any Vs who wish to attend the meetings.
The Thursday Group is responsible for enacting minor policy, the
discussion of current problems and specific crises. This group
gives any V an opportunity to take part in the decision and
policy-making machinery of the CC.

The Executive Director occupies the only paid position in
the CC. The Executive Director oversees the general operation
of the whole CC. He must coordinate all activities, training,
meetings, and other problems which may arise from time to time.

Finally, there is the Board of Directors. This group is
composed of psychologists, other professionals and laymen. Half
of the Board are CC members, and half are community people related to the CC. The responsibility of the Board of Directors
is to create and vote on major policies and oversee financing
of the CC.

Presently, the CC is financed by United Fund, the Wesley
Foundation and other sources. We are hoping to acquire state
and/or Federal funds in the near future.

Publicity for the CC (a responsibility of the Executive
Director) takes the form of public service announcements on the
various radio stations in Tuscaloosa, notices or small public
service advertisements in local newspapers; posters appearing
in Tuscaloosa schools and other conspicuous sites, as well as
live speaking engagements. Trainers or especially well quali-
fied Vs are occasionally asked to speak at school, church or
other social or professional functions. Recently, two Vs video-
taped a program about the CC for educational television.

Moreover, the office of Housing and Urban Development has
selected the Tuscaloosa CC as a model crisis center for the
Southeastern United States.

CRISIS CENTER POLICIES

Our policies and principles of organization and rule making are few,though the ones we do have,we try to adhere to as closely as common sense allows.

Firstly, we attempt to organize the CC in the most parsimonious manner possible; we have as few divisions of labor as necessary. Overlap between different groups within the CC is kept to a minimum, yet cooperation is stressed and usually obtained. Secondly, our rules are created in the interest of assuring smooth, efficient, legitimate, ethical operation of the CC and to guarantee the integrity, anonymity and confidentiality of our callers as well as our Vs. Thirdly, most all rules are put to a vote in our Thursday Meeting. Furthermore, no rule is ironclad. We recognize that there are sometimes exceptional circumstances which necessitate the breaking of a rule. All policies have a built-in margin to provide for human judgment and decision-making in ambiguous situations.

In sum, our organization, policies and rules are governed by our belief that a V's attitude toward volunteer work should be professional. We believe that we have an obligation to our work, to those who direct it, to our colleagues, to those for whom it is done, and to the public.

Following are some of the major policy measures established by the Board of Directors. These policies may be found in the CC's Training Manual, 3rd Edition, October, 1971.

1. The only people permitted in the phone room are trained or in-training Vs, backup personnel, and other individuals with an official relationship with the CC's functioning. Moreover, only the above personnel are permitted to read the logbook. Vs are requested to ask any unknown person to identify himself and if he is not one of the above types of individuals, he is to be politely but firmly asked to leave the phone room. Visitors may stay in our livingroom where they have access to soft drinks, cigarettes and candy in addition to television. Sometimes it is permissable for a V to leave the phone room when he is alone on duty if he leaves the door open or puts the phone in the hallway so it can be heard.

2. All phone calls must be logged in the logbook. Personal incoming calls may be entered as "personal" without further detail.

3. All illegal drugs and alcohol are strictly forbidden in the CC. Individuals under the influence of drugs or alcohol can-

not answer phones. Whether they can remain anywhere in the CC
is still an unresolved issue. If, however, their behavior becomes obnoxious or annoying for any reason, they must be asked
to leave.

4. People who walk into the CC with a crisis should be
treated as the circumstances dictate and in the best judgment of
the V on duty. In any event, the professional backup must be
notified and informed of any decision made. The walk-in cannot
be helped in the phone room. If he calls up first and asks if
he can come to the CC for help, a V, *before* he answers the
caller, must consult the backup and ask for his opinion. If the
backup recommends against a walk-in, the crisis should be dealt
with as best as possible over the phone.

5. Except in an emergency, a maximum of four or five
people should be in the phone room. During a call, silence
should be the rule in the phone room. The V on duty should not
be afraid to ask annoying individuals to quiet down or leave the
phone room.

6. Sometimes it is necessary for Vs to leave the CC to
help a caller in distress. The same rules generally hold as in
policy #4. That is, the V must call the backup on duty at that
time and ask him, *before* the V commits himself either way to the
caller, whether it is appropriate to leave the CC to help the
caller. If the V is the only one on duty, he must call up another
V and ask him to replace himself *before* he leaves the CC. At no
time should the CC be unstaffed. At least *two* Vs must go out on
a crisis call; preferably a male and female. Two females should
not go out on a call alone. The Vs are urged to meet the C in a
public place so as to minimize any danger to the Vs.

7. Except in emergencies, no V should establish a "clientele". That is, he should not allow or encourage a specific
caller to call *only* himself or any particular V. If confronted
with this prospect, a V can inform the caller that *any* V can
handle the callers problem and that a record of the problem is
chronicled in a logbook (confidentially and anonymously) so that
the caller would not have to repeat his problem to a different V.

8. All Vs, when they come on duty, should familiarize themselves with recent logbook entires and any notes left by earlier
Vs that refer to a particular prior crisis or ongoing crisis.

9. The CC discourages non-Vs from sleeping overnight at the
CC. This is especially true in the case of minors and particularly female minors. Violation of this policy might possibly
result in kidnapping charges filed against the CC.

EVALUATION OF CRISIS INTERVENTION SUCCESS: FOLLOW-UP

The question of follow-up and obtaining feedback from Cs about the quality of our service has been heatedly discussed in the past.

Proponents of follow-up, set it as an opportunity to evaluate the effectiveness of our service, a chance to demonstrate concern and interest in the resolution of one's personal crisis, and that since the only source of feedback about the quality of our service is from the caller himself, service improvement requires a follow-up. To get around violations of confidentiality, follow-up would have been carried out only in the case of serious calls, in which callers gave their permission to be contacted again at a later date. The caller would give only a first name, phone number and a time to be called. In turn, the CC would keep the data, of course, strictly confidential. In calling back, the V would not immediately identify himself as representing the CC in case someone other than the original C answered the phone. The caller would be told that his name and phone number would be destroyed after the follow-up was completed.

Opponents of the follow-up issue argued that: 1) if the CC tried to follow-up serious drug problems, some especially suspicious individuals would either immediately hang up, not call again, or still worse, spread the word in the community to the effect that the CC has possibly "sold out to the police", and 2) that word would go around town that the CC does not keep caller's anonymous or confidential; therein possibly rendering the service ineffective.

Other crisis centers around the country were contacted regarding this follow-up issue. Several indicated that callers with drug problems were reluctant to dispense information but that the caller did so if he was in a critical situation. Of four centers contacted, none reported any decrease in drug calls as a function of their follow-up request. However, a V at one center was not sure of this.

As it turned out, the opponents of follow-up emerged victorious. The Tuscaloosa CC does not now, as a result of a vote, officially follow-up any of its calls. We have tried to partially circumvent this problem by allowing a V, in appropriate instances, to occasionally as a C to call back to let us know if and how he resolved his problem. A few callers do call back on their own accord. However, this general kind of feedback is still biased and usually in a positive direction. We appreciate positive feedback, but we would also benefit from negative comments and constructive criticism and suggestions for improving

TUSCALOOSA COMMUNITY CRISIS CENTER

Statistical Data of Calls as of August 28, 1972 based on a
Sample of Every Tenth Call Ranging from Call Number 3,000
Through Call Number 17,000

Average number of calls per day	14
Range of length of calls	0.5 seconds to 6 hours 50 minutes
Shifts	Six 4-hour shifts every day of the year opened Dec. 11, 1970)
Volunteers	60 active men and women
Total number of calls (corrected)	5,458

Type of Call Received	Number	%	Mean Length of Call (minutes)
Miscellaneous	379	30.5	--
Hang-ups, wrong numbers, and silent calls	245	19.7	--
Drugs	74	5.9	13
Boy-girl problems	71	5.7	12
Chronic	70	5.6	16
Information and curious	68	5.4	04
Pregnancy, abortion and Birth control	59	4.7	10
Family	48	3.8	19
Depression	44	3.5	43
Prank	34	2.7	03
Medical	33	2.6	08
Lonely	21	1.7	27
Interpersonal relations	19	1.5	25
Drinking problems	16	1.3	12
Third party	16	1.3	19
Legal	14	1.1	05
Financial	12	1.0	03
Outgoing calls	10	.8	07
Race relations	7	.6	11
Suicide	4	.3	15
Walk-ins	1	.1	25

Total   1,244

our service. Other than the above-mentioned difficulties, no additional problems have been encountered in our effort to compile follow-up data.

QUANTITATIVE ANALYSES OF CRISIS CALLS

Statistical data have been compiled by CC Vs and professional backup personnel. While these data are rather dated, it nevertheless can provide the reader with an idea of the kinds and quantity of calls the CC received in its past. The mean duration of the various kinds of calls have exhibited wide ranges and substantial variability. Moreover, the mean duration of each call provided trainers with a clue to weaknesses in training procedures. For example, the mean duration of "race" calls was a disappointing two minutes. Improved training in this area and bringing such a fact to the attention of the Vs has increased the average length of these calls. Nevertheless, a problem was indicated in the area of race relations. There are very few Black individuals working at the CC. The Tuscaloosa CC positively does not discriminate, indeed has tried to recruit Black Vs and trainers. Unfortunately, due to distance from the CC, often no means of transportation, lack of money and pressing immediate problems in their community, our Black recruitment drive has not been highly successful. Plans for a satellite CC in Tuscaloosa's Black community were never realized. We have no way of accurately assessing how many Blacks call the CC though we fear it to be a disproportionately low number. Recently, the Afro-American Cultural Center of the University of Alabama established its headquarters right next door to the CC. We are trying to solicit Vs from members of that organization.

CONCLUSION

In summary, this paper has briefly outlined the history, purpose, policies, operation, strengths and weaknesses of the Tuscaloosa CC. Our goals for the future include expanding our "walk-in" facilities and phone service, implementing a follow-up program that would not jeopardize the trust and confidence that the Tuscaloosa community presently has in us, as well as hopes to attract more members of the Black community to work with and call on the CC. We welcome the advice, comments and constructive criticism of any other crisis center regarding these or other issues.

In turn, the writer hopes that other crisis centers themselves benefit from this, the story of the Tuscaloosa Community

Crisis Intervention Center.

NOTE: Mr. Stern expressed his indebtedness to the following:
Mr. Chuven, Mr. Lowe, Mr. Thomason and Drs. Dinoff, Miller,
Rivenbark and Rosenberg.

7: EXPERIENTIAL CRISIS TRAINING

All too frequently, according to Dr. Berman, methods used in training paraprofessionals to man emergency telephone crisis centers consist of superficial and boring formal talks prepared by the professional for the non-professional. Dr. Berman strongly advocates active experiential and organized specialized training permitting students to model effective work behavior.

From these pedigogical preferences evolved the BEST method (an immodest acronym) for training crisis workers, emphasizing behavioral, experiential and simulation techniques. Simulating aspects of intrapersonal crisis permits the worker to have an experiential understanding of the psychological aspects of crisis. The person in crisis can relate to the worker personally experientially and existentially; these ways of relating are normally precluded by traditional patient-therapist diagnostic perspectives. For Berman, crisis involves a problem solving process in which the experience of success and failure produce emotionally similar feeling states. Through simulation exercises individual hotline workers are brought to the point of experiencing and understanding the situations likely to be represented by their clientel.

The second half of this chapter outlines a set of exercises which sample the domain of the potential simulation techniques, each reflecting the value system espoused by Dr. Berman. Some may find these techniques suited to immediate use; others will see them as illustrations which are suggestive of other techniques matched to the individual training needs. Dr. Berman's training model should have wide application over the range of crisis intervention tasks.

While these exercises represent an experiential and existential bias, they are open to rigorous logical-positivist evaluation. Dr. Berman emphasizes the importance of the articulation of target behaviors and the development of criteria for evaluation of training. It is in this sense that Dr. Berman's contribution is an advance rather than a diversion in crisis intervention conceptualization.

EXPERIENTIAL TRAINING FOR CRISIS INTERVENTION

Alan L. Berman

American University

BACKGROUND

Since the opening of the first Suicide Prevention Center in Los Angeles in 1958, the number of suicide prevention, crisis intervention, telephone "hotline," and free clinic services manned and operated by paraprofessionals has proliferated at an astronomic rate. The professional mental health community, for the most part, has attempted to respond to these developments positively; offering support, consultation and training to a wide variety of these new helping agents. The motivation for this professional response is, indeed, complex; but, clearly derives, in part, from the perceived need for these services, from the manpower demands confronting the helping professions, and from a concern that if these services are to be truly helpful, training is essential.

In the rush to train this new manpower, however, the professional community has behaved much like the client in crisis, *i.e.*, by falling back on old, well-tried, but presently inapplicable modes of coping and adaptation. What the professional has learned through several years of graduate education suddenly, and miraculously, must now be condensed and communicated in as few as six hours of training. Rather than adapt training to achieve reachable goals, much effort has been expended in attempting to make "junior professionals" quickly. The models maintained for most training programs for paraprofessional-operated crisis intervention services are not only inapplicable, but also rather outmoded and sterile. Considerable time is spent, for example, on lectures - on suicide, drugs, depression, crisis theory, etc. While these presentations of informational content are, no doubt, important and essential, the most necessary, reachable, productive and yet ignored training need for these services is in "listening", "empathy," and "behavioral change" skills.

Even for those training programs which do concern themselves with training for the "good listener", however, training goals (and therefore methods) are often couched in such nonoperationalized globalisms as "listening to the whole person," and the like. As an all too frequent result, the only training designed and used to develop these skills is that of role-playing and its variations. More importantly, this is often the only "experiential" counterpart to the more generally used didactic training formats. Where attention is paid to the development of sensitivity and empathy among paraprofessional workers, it usually is in the form of sensitivity training sessions offered to these students. Here again, while helpful, these formats are used most often as adjunctive training devices to compliment more traditional (didactic) methods of teaching and do not pay specific attention to the goals and skills necessary to be a paraprofessional helper.

The art and science of "training" in helping skills is still in its infancy. Research studies of the effectiveness of various training approaches most commonly result in only gross generalizations, *e.g.*, that *some* training is better than no training at all (*c.f.*, Carkhuff and Truax, 1965). Thoreson (1969) has argued, additionally, that a common problem encountered in these studies is that a single global criterion (index) of training effectiveness has been used, thus making results misleading. The problem boils down to the question of whether training objectives can be operationally stated and whether identified constructs are teachable (Danish, 1971). Considering the diverse roles that paraprofessionals are expected to perform, the utility of identifying a basic set of skills which can be taught readily and applied across a variety of potential functions is obvious.

The development and application of innovative training models both to non-traditional criteria and within grossly altered temporal conditions presents a unique challenge to the consultant-trainer. Practically all of the existing crisis services have developed their own and often idiosyncratic (to service and to trainer) procedures for developing the skills of their own crisis workers. Nearly all training programs not only ignore the factors stated above, but, in addition, pay little attention to accepted principles of learning. Where training (and learning) should be active, it is often passive (lecture presentations). Where training (and learning) should be experiential, it is often abstract (theories and dynamics). Where training (and learning) should be step-wise and sequential, it is more often than not haphazard and unsystematic. Where training (and learning) should be open to observation it is more often of the "do as I say I do" variety, rather than that of the professional "modeling" the proper responses (Berman and McCarthy, 1971).

As a result of this lack of an appropriate training model, and specific training techniques, a reversing trend is becoming evident with many paraprofessional services closing their doors and hanging up their phones in greater and greater numbers. Some might argue that these occurrences represent the burning out of a "fad" and this cannot be counter-argued. It is, however, unfortunate that a fad, if constructive, cannot be maintained. There is a good deal of evidence that paraprofessional crisis intervention services serve a real mental health need, and that their disappearance would be a backward step for the community mental health movement. Part of these failures, I firmly believe, may most parsimoniously be explained as a response to the failure of the professional community to develop and offer adequate models of training for these services.

My own work in the area of paraprofessional crisis intervention services began in January, 1970 with the development and implementation of a student-operated, campus-based, crisis intervention telephone service. The model for this service is based on the premise that the professional's major contribution to a paraprofessionally operated crisis intervention service is as trainer and consultant (McCarthy and Berman, 1971; Berman and McCarthy, 1972). The models of training which I and Dr. McCarthy have employed have evolved out of our experiences with this service and are undergoing continual modification. As we have observed continual modifications in professional training (c.f., Pottharst, 1970; Leventhal, 1971) and the use of a variety of models and techniques of training, e.g., the use of videotape (Berger, 1970), simulation (Corsini, 1966), and combinations of methods (Ivey, et al., 1968); we have adapted a variety of techniques for use in our consultation with our own and other services. At present, the training model developed for the American University service includes only about four hours of didactic material (although there are, additionally, a variety of required and suggested reading materials available for students) out of a total of approximately 30 hours of initial training. The bulk of the training focuses on behavioral, experiential, and simulation techniques (which we have labelled the B.E.S.T. system) for training students. Our belief in this type of model has recently been substantiated, in part, by research reported by Perino (1971). He found that of four methods of training, basic helping skills and experiential models of training were consistently superior to traditional lecture formats with paraprofessional trainees, using five criterion measures.

The purpose of this paper is to describe several of the experiential training devices (modules) currently used in our training program. The goals of these exercises are based on the beliefs outlined above (e.g., active, self-involved learning), as well as a belief that through simulation-self-awareness exercises, such as these, the trainee may invest himself in the learning process as a participant-learner.

Furthermore, as any student of Abnormal Psychology can well recall his first experiences with what is commonly referred to as the "medical student's syndrome" (that peculiar malady, which for a time convinces us that we are surely schizophrenic; or, perhaps, brain damaged; or, perchance, this week, a "true" obsessive-compulsive), the study of human behavior by behaving humans is not an abstract phenomenon. Because human emotions are universal, we are able to experience the response and process of another person's pain or joy. As effective communication depends on a shared field of common experience between the communication's source and destination, training in listening skills must necessitate the trainee's broadened awareness of his own experiences. Through analogy, metaphor, fantasy, and the lessons of the medical student's syndrome, mental health trainers can stimulate both an experiential and active understanding of learning material. More importantly, through creative training approaches, creative learning and risk-taking is modeled, and, therefore, may occur among trainees. Instead of learning to play "junior shrink" or to mimic Carl Rogers, in effect to be what they are not, student trainees may learn to maximize and actualize their potential to be what they are: sensitive, human, and responsive. As a learning model, this approach mirrors what Proshansky (1972) has recently argued for in all forms of undergraduate education:

> We have failed to give (undergraduates) ....
> a curriculum that is educationally significant. By
> *significance*, I mean a course designed in a way that
> deals with the particular issue, problem, or phenomenon in terms of a psychological approach. A
> psychological approach is one way to understand why
> a problem occurs and what might be done about it.
> Its purpose is not to provide the student with all
> the existing theories, the conflicting findings, and
> the tantalizing jargon, but to help him understand,
> think about, and relate his own experience to the
> problem or phenomenon under consideration. (p. 209).

EXPERIENTIAL TRAINING MODULES

The methods described below owe considerably to the learnings of encounter/sensitivity groups and game theory. The specific exercises have been begged, borrowed, stolen, and/or created for purposes not necessarily analogous to those being related herein.

Each exercise is introduced and discussed in terms of the underlying rationale or premise for its application to crisis intervention training. Common and relevant points for discussion follow each specific method. As a final note, these exercises are presented as examples of a varity of applicable experiential tools. No determined sequence or coordination between the specific exercises discussed in the following presentation is intended.

Exercise: Crisis as Transition

Premise. Caplan (1964) views a crisis as a transitional period, presenting to the individual in crisis an opportunity for personality growth. The transitional state is often characterized by feelings of pain or disequilibrium from which is sought a return to a state of no pain, homeostasis, or equilibrium.

Method. "Close your eyes...relax...and think about how, in what way(s), you are currently or were recently experiencing some transition in your life (*e.g.*, a change of job, change of academic major, graduation, change of boy or girl friend, etc.)... Focus on your feelings as you recall and experience this transitional period. Develop the conflicts you sense.... Be aware, as you do this, of your feelings and your body"... (5 minutes). "Now choose a partner (dyads) and share this experience with them..." (10 minutes).

Group Discussion. Elicit the feelings and conflicts expressed. Note especially the sense of pain, disequilibrium, fears of taking risks, signs of obsessional indecision, signs of acute anxiety expressed as concomitants of the pre-transitional state.

Exercise: Crisis and Creativity

Premise. The process of crisis resolution is similar to and demands the availability of the coallescence of existing behavioral repertoires in creative problem solving. Creativity and crisis resolution share a common beginning point - a blockage of effective problem solving skills and the concurrent experience of pain, discomfort, and impotence. The person becomes upset, feels helpless and ineffectual in the face of an insoluable problem. The usual homeostatic, direct problem-solving mechanisms do not work. Every crisis represents a novel situation in which novel forces, both internal and external, are involved (Caplan, 1964).

Method. "Close your eyes...relax...get by yourself. Take the next few minutes to get into yourself. Think about yourself as a 'creative' person. Get at those past and present creative moments you have experienced. These may be among those areas we usually associate with creativity, *e.g.,* art, music, writing, etc. - but, even more importantly, among equally as creative experiences, for example, in interpersonal relationships, fantasies, etc.... Try to arrive at your 'most creative moment' -that peak experience or time you can recall when you were most proud of a particular creative achievement.... Develop this moment and try to recall your feelings, thoughts, etc., as you recapture your creative process...." (5 minutes). "Now choose and share with a partner your experiences during this exercise" (5-10 minutes).

Group Discussion. Note the similarities between the expressions of this and the preceeding exercise: the sense of pain which appears equally strong in achieving a creative moment, the helplessness and impotence prior to breakthrough, etc. Furthermore, elicit the methods of integration and production involved in problem resolution, the seeking of interpersonal support, the need to break out of habitual response patterns, etc.

Exercise: On Pathology Focus vs. Strength Identification

Premise. The individual in crisis has tunnel vision - a selective scanning of his relationship to his world which momentarily has blurred his perceptions. He sees weaknesses where there exists the potential for strength. Even when either exogenous or endogenous conditions are not such as to maximize the individual's tendency to be self-depreciatory, feel helpless, etc., there exists a cultural tendency in our society which says, in effect,: If you think well of yourself, shut up, lest you be seen as conceited, egocentric, etc....Thus, while Bellak and Small (1965) emphasize the use of reassurance and identification of ego-strengths as primary components in effective brief psychotherapy, even the normal, healthy, not-in-crisis individual may "tune out" messages of compliment, reassurance, and strength identification. How often do we hear "how uncomfortable I feel when someone compliments me." If this is the response of a healthy ego, what then can we suppose about the ego which is sensed as helpless and ineffectual. As difficult as it is to hear the positive, it is equally as difficult to communicate the positive.

Method. (Pair trainees in dyads). "For the next six minutes (6') each of you will have the opportunity to tell each other how you feel about yourself. Each of you will have three minutes (3') to talk and three minutes (3') to listen. As one of you speaks, the other is to not respond in any way. Decide which of you will speak first. I will start you and tell you when your 3' are up. You should then switch roles, *i.e.*, the listener will then talk, the first talker will then listen."

"There is but one rule to be adhered to. Your messages communicated during your 3' of talking to your partner are restricted to only good things about yourself (*e.g.*, 'I am smart'; 'I feel strong,'....). Negative statements are not allowed; nor are qualifiers, *e.g.*, 'maybe,' 'but,' 'except when,'.... That is, do not allow yourself to say 'I am pretty, but I wish my nose were less crooked'."

Group Discussion. Focus on feelings of perplexity, impotence, etc., experienced by trainees in attempting to follow these rules but for only three minutes. Note the tendencies to qualify, to become silent or hesitant to verbalize.

Follow-up. After a brief discussion (5') ask the partners to spend two minutes apiece sharing what their partner communicated to them (positive self-statements) during the original 3 minute sharing. Each dyad member is to say "I...", filling in with what was heard, but communicated as if he were his partner.

Group Discussion. Note how few of those positive messages originally communicated were really heard; or, if heard, how they might have been misinterpreted by the listener. Note, also, how the second (to speak) partner may have heard less than the other member of the dyad, due to his concentration on (rehearsal of) what he/she was going to say when his/her turn to speak came. Discuss how often we have the tendency to get caught up in the "appropriate thing to say" ("Now, how would Rogers respond to that..."), and, in the process, stop hearing what is communicated to us.

Exercise: The Risk of the "Want" vs. the "Should"

Premise. Crisis intervention seeks the resolution of conflict. The potential for change (conflict resolution) exists within us all. The unwillingness to take the risk to change, *i.e.*, to grow, however, is more often than not the blockade to successful intervention. The risk, in Gestalt terms, exists between the want and the should; the latter, being a surrender of personal control, presumably to more powerful others. Cohn (1968) has described this exercise as a "therapeutic game for therapists, patients, and other people."

Method. "For ten minutes, I must do what I want to. I must check out every moment what I am doing (including body and mental activity) and whether I am really still doing what I want to and, if not, change to what I want to do.

"The rule is not I must do what I feel like doing, but what I want to do. What I 'want to' includes my judgment as well as my impulses: *i.e.*, if I feel like smashing an object, I must check whether I want to follow the impulse which I know will destroy this object, then check whether I would rather vent my feeling now and not have this object thereafter, or whether I would sufficiently enjoy smashing it to take the loss of the object in my stride.

"In my checking it is important to include the awareness of messages from my body. I might have the fantasy that I want to dance, but my body may signal that I am tired now and what I really want is to have a fantasy of dancing. The opposite may be true; I might think that dancing is silly, but my body may want to dance. I then have to make a decision: Which is it that I want? And the decision may come effortlessly by itself within a few seconds, or a third idea may pop up and ring the bell of 'this is it'."

Group Discussion. The clearest experience here is one of conflict, indecision, obsessional immobilization, anxiety, or panic. The game smacks of self-indulgence. Trainees freeze in the hope of permission to be/do what they want. When behavior (doing) occurs, it often has a child-like, regressed (in the service of the ego?) quality so analogous to the process of creative problem solving. The difficulty of doing what one wants teaches an acceptance of or appreciation of a client's resistance to change.

On Empathizing With Drug Crises

Premise. A history of drug use and personal experience with a "bad trip" are not necessary to be able to empathize, understand and respond to the trip. Yet, frequently, the client in panic engenders panic in the helper. Novice telephone workers have often made remarks to this trainer such as: "Drug crises scare me. I would have to give such a call over to another worker if one came in during my shift."

Method. Trainees are asked to recall and focus on a "bad" (non-drug related) experience they have had. After sufficient opportunity for personal reflection, each trainee is asked to label their memory with some adjective or phrase that describes

their feelings, thoughts, or behaviors during this "bad" experience. These, then, are verbalized to the group. (The trainer
may choose to write these on a blackboard or poster paper for
all to see).

Trainees who have experienced a bad drug experience are
asked to call out labelling phrases or adjectives describing
their experiences.

Group Discussion. The similarities between all types of
"bad experiences" will be designated and the parallels drawn
easily (*e.g.*, "loss of control," "powerless," "panic," "helplessness," "will it ever end," etc.) for "straights" to realize
that "bad trips" are not necessarily just drug induced experiences.

Death Awareness Experience

Premise. Death fantasies are common among mentally healthy
individuals. A sensitivity to one's own feelings about death
may prevent the negative intrusion of these feelings (*e.g.*, moralizing or anxiety interference) into the helping interaction
with the suicidal client.

Method. The procedure and results of this exercise have
been described in detail elsewhere (Berman, 1972). Trainees
are asked to write down their responses to the following: 1) were
you to know that you have but one more day to live, how would you
spend your last day?, 2) at what age do you expect your own death
will come?, 3) how do you expect to die?, 4) what were your experiences (feelings, thoughts, etc.) during this exercise?

Trainees are then directed to share their experiences with
other trainees (in dyads) and, if they wish, their specific responses. A large group discussion then follows. If possible
follow up data (further behaviors, thoughts, etc.) is recommended to facilitate the working through of any lingering effects of
this exercise on participants.

Discussion. Similarities between death fantasies and relevant knowledge about actual, attempted, threatened and simulated
suicide acts (and notes) are easily connected. (*c.f.*, Berman,
1972).

CONCLUSION

The list of potential simulation training exercises is as long as the trainer's realm of imagination is broad. Numerous communication exercises are described in the professional and lay literature and any experience is applicable if made so. The benefits subsidiary to those already outlined which accrue from an experiential approach to training are many. Foremost is the sense of shared common experience and its positive effects on the training group's morale which result from active, interpersonal learning. Also, each of these exercises trains and supports self-disclosure and "on target" communication, skills which are very necessary to the ultimate effectiveness of the crisis interventionist. Goals become more consistent with the expectations; content becomes subsidiary to process; and trainees learn to think, to risk, to share, and to be what they are: experiencing human beings.

REFERENCES

Bellak, L. & Small, L. *Emergency psychotherapy and brief psychotherapy.* N.Y.: Grune & Stratton, 1965.

Berger, M. M. *Videotape techniques in psychiatric training and
treatment.* N.Y.: Bruner-Mazel, 1970.

Berman, A. L. Crisis interventionists and death awareness: An
exercise for training in suicide prevention. *Journal of
Crisis Intervention,* 1972, *4,* 47-52.

Berman, A. L. & McCarthy, B. W. The university counseling center
as a training-consultation center. Presented at the meeting
of the American Psychological Association, Washington, D.C.,
September, 1971.

Berman, A. L. & McCarthy, B. W. Curriculum relevance and community mental health. *Journal of College Student Personnel,*
1972, *13,* 77-78.

Caplan, G. *Principles of preventive psychiatry.* N.Y.: Basic
Books, 1964.

Carkhuff, R. R. & Truax, C. B. Training in counseling and psychotherapy: An evaluation of an integrated didactic and experiential approach. *Journal of Consulting Psychology,* 1965,
29, 333-336.

Cohn, R. C. "I must do what I want to". *Voices,* 1968, *4,* 29-33.

Corsini, R. J. *Roleplaying in psychotherapy: A manual.* Chicago:
Aldine, 1966.

Danish, S. J. The basic helping skills program: A proposed model
for training paraprofessionals. Presented at the meeting
of the American Psychological Association, Washington, D.C.,
September, 1971.

Ivey, A. E., Normington, D. J., Miller, C. D., Morrill, W. H., &
Haase, R. F. Microcounseling and attending behavior: An
approach to prepracticum counselor training. *Journal of
Counseling Psychology,* 1968, *15,* Monograph, No. 5.

Leventhal, A. M. The Washington Free Clinic - a training model.
Presented at the workshop on manpower innovations in mental
health crisis intervention services, The American University,
Washington, D.C., January, 1971.

McCarthy, B. W. & Berman, A. L. The development of a student operated crisis center. *Personnel and Guidance Journal*, 1971, *49*, 523-528.

Perino, A. R. A comparison of four methods of training para-professional counselors. Presented at the meeting of the American Psychological Association, Washington, D.C., September, 1971.

Pottharst, E. E. To renew vitality and provide a challenge in training - the California School of Professional Psychology. *Professional Psychology*, 1970, *1*, 123-130.

Proshansky, H. For what are we training our graduate students? *American Psychologist*, 1972, *27*, 205-212.

Simon, R. The paraprofessionals are coming! The paraprofessionals are coming! *The Clinical Psychologist*, 1971, *24*.

Thoreson, C. E. Relevance and research in counseling. *Review of Educational Research*, 1969, *39*, 264-282.

8:    STRATEGIES FOR EVALUATION

Emergency telephone services are one of the newer developments on the mental health scene. Their organization, function,
and effectiveness have been subject to wide and mixed reviews.
Several questions have been raised, but left unanswered: do
hotlines tap new populations or do they represent alternate or
additional service to those normally ordinarily utilizing the
more traditional services? Does the Hotline create its own
need? Does the availability of places to call itself determine
the need and the use of such facilities? If the need for these
services developed as a result of the increasing complexity of
urban living, what should be the essential services provided by
the Hotline? Should there be training standards for all workers?
Should hotlines be regulated and controlled by mental health
professionals?

Despite the faddish popularity of these new emergency services some are underutilized. Further, many of them suffer from
poor quality of training and poorly defined functions. These
hotlines may be better serving the personal needs of the people
manning them than they are serving needs of the community.
References on the diversity and extent of hotline services can
be found in Brennan (1972).

In this short chapter, Bleach reviews research strategies
that can be applied to hotline and other emergency telephone
services for evaluation of their effectiveness. As pointed out
in the chapter by Berman, single criterion measures for evaluating complex performances are destined to be unsatisfactory.
Bleach suggests a number of alternative assessment strategies
including the use of unobtrusive measures and simple demographic
records, as well as the establishment of more rigorous research
programs. She discusses the dangers and risks of intruding on
a service which depends on confidentiality for its credibility
and is often characterized by the reluctance of workers to open
themselves to scrutiny. Her solution featured an analogue paradigm involving simulated phone calls and subsequent evaluation
of the quality of information and therapeutic value of the
worker's response to the caller (Bleach & Claiborn, in press).

The analogue method, in its variations, can provide an effective, relatively nonthreating device for examining many aspects of service-delivery, without the necessity of involving service users, themselves, in the research design. Such techniques can be employed to determine the quality of workers training and to define the range of worker behavior in response to callers with varying kinds of problems. This kind of strategy is least likely to be sabotaged by passive-aggressive or active maneuvers on the part of staff and does the least damage to confidentiality and trust with the community.

As some of the excitement over hotline begins to wane, presumably only the more effective services will survive. Evaluative research may help by setting of service standards to obtain community and financial support for quality programs.

The range of emergency telephone service functions continue to be defined by practice. Conceptual models, criteria for evaluation and operating "policy" have lagged far behind. Critical research should help build a badly needed knowledge base.

REFERENCES

Bleach, G., & Claiborn, W. L.   Initial evaluation of hotline telephone crisis centers. *Community Mental Health Journal,* 1974, In press.

Brennan, J. *The use of the telephone for hotline services and medical care.* Research Memo #71, Shepard and Enoch Pratt Hospital, Towson, Md. 1972.

STRATEGIES FOR EVALUATION OF HOTLINE

TELEPHONE CRISIS CENTERS

Gail Bleach

University of Maryland

The growing number of crisis centers which offer intervention services via the telephone is a readily observable fact.
In the Washington area alone to date there are at least fifteen
Hotline crisis services established by hospitals, mental health
associations, colleges, and others. These Hotline services
share the following defining characterists: 1) they operate
during week-end and evening hours when traditional helping agencies are closed, 2) they are staffed by nonprofessional or paraprofessional workers, 3) they accept calls from anyone in the
community and on any topic the caller presents, 4) they offer
advice, information, and referral services, and 5) they allow
their clients to remain anonymous.

Research on the effectiveness of these services poses special problems all centering around the issue of how the most
informative, well-controlled research can be done with the least
disruption to the crisis service. This paper will discuss a
number of data collection methods and related criterion measures which might be used in studying the effectiveness of Hotline services. Emphasis will be placed on the expected impact
on and reception of these methods by the crisis services.

Perhaps the simplest and least disruptive outcome data to
collect is demographic data. Most Hotlines are presently recording such information as: 1) number of calls received, 2)
length of the calls, 3 time and date of the call, 4) problem
presented, and 5) disposition of the call. This information
can answer certain questions about how a Hotline service can
most efficiently be run. For example, the problems most frequently encountered or the time of day calls most frequently
occur can be tabulated. Based on these data, it might be suggested that, for instance, more training be given in pregnancy
counseling than in draft counseling because pregnancy problem

calls are heard substantially more often. As another example, more workers need to be scheduled for the afternoon shift than the morning shift because considerably more calls are received during the later shift. Hotlines can also gather some minimal information about the general effectiveness of their services from demographic data. For instance, based on a comparison of Hotline statistics, it is reasonable to assume that well-publicized Hotlines that are receiving less than one hundred calls per week are handling callers poorly.

The main advantage of using this kind of data is that data collection is minimally intrusive to the Hotline services. However, even here, resistance of Hotline workers should not be underestimated. The idea of any evaluation is threatening to a service that has not yet been integrated into the traditional mental health services network and that still needs to convince taxpayers or college administrators that it is deserving of funds. Also, filling out statistical forms often seems irrelevant and bothersome to Hotline workers who would prefer to spend their time on the telephone. Thus, in instituting even simple data collection procedures, researchers should expect careful scrutiny by the personnel involved and should be prepared to explain the benefits that the Hotlines might derive from the research.

The main disadvantage with using only demographic data to measure effectiveness is the criterion problem. Knowing that a Hotline receives 250 calls per day, for example is clearly not a sufficient criteria for calling it an effective service. Other variables like the size of the youth population or the number of other Hotlines in the area influence the number of calls received. All demographic data share this difficulty of not controlling relevant variables and therefore provide suggestive but not conclusive answers to effectiveness questions.

At the other end of the continuum from demographic data are rigorous but highly intrusive experimental designs. This kind of procedure might involve asking Hotline callers for their names or a place they can be reached and then contacting them at a later date. Subjective feelings of the callers about the helpfulness of a Hotline would be used as the primary effectiveness criterion. Callers might be asked such questions as:
"Did talking to Hotline make you feel better?"
"Did the information provided turn out to be useful to you?"
"Did you contact any agencies or other resources to which you were referred by Hotline?"
"Do you think you will have some ideas about what to do the next time this problem arises?"
A more objective procedure where the nature and seriousness of the presenting problem were evaluated (perhaps by a rating

system) at the time of the original call and again at a later date could also be designed.

The advantages of this procedure are apparent; effectiveness could be measured through contact with the individuals whom Hotline is supposed to affect. As well as providing evaluative data, this design could provide some precise information about possible ways to improve Hotline services. For example, data about which referral sources prove most helpful should lead to a greater number of referrals to those sources.

Disadvantages of a procedure that directly contacts Hotline users center around the potential impact of the research on the users. There is a general feeling among Hotline personnel that a substantial proportion of their growth can be attributed to their policy of anonymity for the caller. This promise of no feedback to either parents or law enforcement agencies distinguishes them from many traditional mental health services. It may be as important in attracting the youth population as either Hotline's ease of accessibility (via the telephone) or its hours of operation (at night and on week-ends), factors which crisis intervention theories propose to explain Hotline's appeal. For this reason as well as for the general concerns about evaluations discussed above, any procedure which interferes with the policy of anonymity and which therefore may lower trust or confidence in the Hotline service is likely to meet with serious difficulty in securing staff cooperation. This is not to suggest that such research should not be done but only that it should be planned with full knowledge of the problems involved.

Between the two procedures discussed thus far are the procedures which attempt to balance selection of maximally useful criterion with concern for interference in services rendered. One way to accomplish this is to evaluate worker effectiveness as the author did in a recent study (Bleach & Claiborn, in press). The procedure used trained undergraduates posing as Hotline users. These students called a sample of Hotlines in the Washington area and presented standardized stories about problems they were having. Calls were taped and then rated on a series of scales which assessed worker skills along two dimensions--counseling skills and information-giving skills. Counseling skills were rated on the Truax-Carkhuff scales of empathy, warmth, and genuineness. Information scales which were written by the author provided an assessment of accuracy of information, number and quality of alernatives, and number and quality of referrals presented.

Findings of the study provide some data about effectiveness and about potential improvements services can implement. One finding, for example, was that worker skills do not measurably improve as a function of length of time worked. This suggests that effectiveness could be increased by teaching workers to evaluate and learn from the calls that they answer. Another finding of interest was that one of the four Hotlines included in the study demonstrated higher skill levels on a number of the scales than the other Hotlines. This Hotline had the most rigorous training program which placed special emphasis on instruction in counseling skills.

One main advantage of this procedure was that promises of confidentiality to callers were not violated since no data were collected about actual callers. Another advantage was that it allowed for experimental control of variables such as presenting problem and caller differences and thus permitted comparisons across Hotlines. The main limitation of the study centered around the choice of criteria; the assumption that quality of worker skills was adequately measured by the scales employed was not experimentally validated.

The need for balancing intrusiveness with experimental rigor when selecting criterion measures is not unique to Hotline research. Other crisis intervention research faces the problem to some degree. Suicide prevention centers, for example, confront the issues of anonymity as well as concerns about the possible dangers of a follow-up on a suicidal individual. Yet, it is difficult for suicide prevention centers to know if they are saving lives, which is the ultimate effectiveness criterion, without having the names of their callers and doing a follow-up check.

In sum, research on the effectiveness of crisis intervention services can have important theoretical and practical implications. Sound methodological studies designed with a knowledge of the special problems involved in researching crisis intervention services are much needed at the present time.

REFERENCES

Bleach, G. & Claiborn, W.   Initial evaluation of Hotline Telephone Crisis Centers.   *Community Mental Health Journal,*
1974, in press.

IV: INNOVATIVE SERVICES

We have no doubt that across the country there are hund-
reds of innovative programs falling under the crisis intervention rubric. Some incorporate research designs which provide
meaningful information about their impact, others are justified
solely by the Zeitgeist. Programs can develop from local community support, theory put to practice, or "seat-of-the pants"
reactions to immediate need.

The four chapters in this section present four radically
different areas of "crisis": transition from the mental hospital
to home, management of mourning, the crisis of the bad drug trip,
and the multiple crisis family. They also differ widely on the
level of intervention from direct professional service, the
training of natural help givers, the use of natural 'gate-
keeping' non-professional, to the involvement of ever available
college students.

These chapters might be considered a "Latin Square" assort-
ment of strategy, manpower, and focus. The remaining cells of
potential crisis work are easily generated and the matrix can be
completed by the program developer.

On another level of analysis, these chapters reveal implicit models of crisis intervention and of human behavior which
dictate the thrust of the program. This is particularly evident and well articulated in the chapter by Jaffe.

This chapter by Freitag, Blechman and Berck illustrates
a number of unique and interesting issues. A particularly noteworthy point relates to the way in which the client population
was reached. The majority of crisis intervention efforts cited
in this book and elsewhere have relied upon the potential client
to initiate the relationship with the help-giving agency. This
strategy may be inevitably dictated in many cases, because crises are often precipitated by events which crisis workers could
not predict or readily identify. There are, however, certain
situations which the worker might readily suppose would engend-
er crises, and where efforts to reach out to those likely to be
effected may be appropriate. Freitag and associates deal with
one such situation, the extrusion of the mental patient back
into the community. Their work illustrates the possibility of
having the crisis intervenor position himself so as to provide
supportive resources before environmental stresses lead to a
failure of adaptation. Such a strategy may be particularly
appropriate when, as in the present case, the client population already has a history of psychosocial failure and consequent community exclusion.

A second intriguing issue raised in this chapter concerns
the compatibility of service delivery and research. Freitag
et al. were able to meet most of the criteria for rigorous research while, at the same time, providing a potentially useful
service. The key factor may have been that the experiment
and treatment goals of the project were united from their inception. The problems of assessing existing service systems
after the fact may be so great as to virtually preclude the
collection of useful data.

A third point of special interest concerns the efforts to
assess the effects of varying the degree to which the client
affected the college student crisis worker. Under one condition the students met with discharged patients with the mutual
understanding that the patient would partially determine the
student's grade by evaluating his performance; in the other
condition the patient did not evaluate the helper for grading

purposes. Although the results of the study did not show differential effects under the two conditions, the basic notion
may yet warrant further study. The possibility exists that
efforts to collect follow-up data on any crisis intervention
might actually benefit clients by giving them a choice to perceive the helping relationship as one in which they are not
powerless to affect the help-giver and in which they have a
competent role (see chapter by Korner).

Although Freitag *et al.* failed to demonstrate that the
intervention would effect gross measures of the post-discharge
adaptation of patients, the authors state several possible reasons for this failure. A major determinant may have been the
selection and training of helpers (see papers by Bleach, Berman,
and Sebolt for further consideration of these issues). The
authors note that the college students were rather unlike the
patients with whom they worked and that the students received
no extensive preparation for their helping role. It is at
least possible that matching helpers to clients or training
helpers more effectively might have altered the measured outcome
of their interventions.

COLLEGE STUDENTS AS COMPANION AIDES TO NEWLY-RELEASED

PSYCHIATRIC PATIENTS

Gilbert Freitag   Elaine Blechman

University of California   University of Maryland

Los Angeles   College Park

and Philip Berck

University of California, Los Angeles

There are several critical tasks of adjustment facing persons returning to community life following lengthy institutional confinement. These include securing adequate housing and financial support, arranging for travel and companionship, and arriving at a new self-appraisal that reflects one's autonomous noninstitutionalized status. These tasks are particularly acute for the psychiatric patient (Camp and Onnenebo, 1968; Freeman and Simmons, 1963; Stewart, Selkirk, and Aydiaha, 1969). Effectiveness in performing the tasks at re-entry can determine the difference between successful adaptation to community life or recidivism (Purvis and Miekunins, 1970).

The period immediately following hospital release was the focus of the present study. Viewed as an "emotionally hazardous situation" (Klein and Lindemann, 1961), it was thought that the ex-patient would experience this time as a period of emotional crisis to the extent he felt an imbalance between the difficulty and importance of the tasks encountered at release and the resources immediately available to him (Caplan, 1964).

The central task facing the psychiatric patient upon hospital release was viewed as effecting a transition between two social roles: the role of a mentally "sick" person, almost entirely dependent on hospital staff for a wide range of personal needs (Levinson and Gallagher, 1961), and the role of a "mentally healthy" individual, capable of functioning autonomously in meeting one's own needs. In the latter role the person must

118

interact in a variety of ways with an expanded set of significant others--family, friends, social agents (*e.g.*, employer,
landlord, pharmacist), and social agencies (*e.g.*, department of
social welfare, office of unemployment, department of motor
vehicles). The two roles differ in important respects. It was
expected that where they compete in their demands on the patient, he will have difficulty in making the transition (Sarbin,
1970).

The psychological tasks involved in successful role transition have been conceptualized elsewhere (Newton and Brown, 1968)
as involving at least three sets of functions:

1) developing new role behaviors to meet expectations of
home and community. For the ex-mental patient this could include getting a prescription filled, a check cashed, a driver's
license renewed.

2) developing new interpersonal relationships and modify-
ing the old; *e.g.*, meeting new people, developing relationships with persons that can support new efforts at adaptation
rather than old inadequacies, despite unfavorable and often
hostile or dehumanizing public attitudes toward the mentally
ill.

3) management and desirable expression of feelings; *e.g.*,
handling the feelings of loss and insecurity at leaving the pro-
tected environment of the hospital, accommodating to the feelings of increased responsibility, independence, and isolation.

To this can be added a fourth:

4) developing new cognitions of situation and self; *e.g.*,
learning to recognize alternative ways of interacting socially
which are more satisfying and effective in achieving desired
ends, recognizing strengths as well as weaknesses and developing a sense of competency and self-worth.

In the mental patient, the behavioral, social, emotional
and cognitive skills necessary for effective functioning in
these areas may be absent or unavailable. This may be related
to a variety of factors, including his premorbid level of adjustment, the disturbance itself, his hospital role, and the
amount and availability of outside resources at the time of
hospital release. It was the central aim of this project to
develop a program of aftercare which would remedy this last
factor, and provide the ex-mental patient with an additional
human resource to aid in the transition. It was hoped such a
service would reduce the hazardous aspects of transition and
thereby maximize successful efforts at community adjustment.

While it appears that after-care services are essential to the prevention of further disability and subsequent rehospitalization, the need for such services far outweighs the availability of trained personnel who could best provide it. The use of college undergraduates in meeting the critical manpower shortage in the mental health field has already been widely documented. Numerous projects report that with a minimal amount of selection and training college students are successful and effective in performing a variety of sub-professional helping functions with a range of psychiatric populations (*e.g.*, Cowen, Zax, and Laird, 1966; Guerney, 1970). This has been particularly true with chronic hospitalized patients (Holzberg, Knapp, and Turner, 1967; Umbarger, Morrison, Dalsimer, and Breggin, 1962). To date, the college student has not been utilized in any systematic way in providing after-care. It was a second aim of this study to create a new role for the college undergraduate, one of companion aide to newly released psychiatric patients.

A final aim of the study was to utilize the helping relationship students would create with patients as an opportunity to examine certain social-psychological variables and processes thought to influence the nature of the relationship. The intent was to create a community laboratory, not only for program evaluation, but also for investigations of a theoretical or experimental nature. The genuine interactions of student and patient extended over a specific time period was viewed as a unique context within which to conduct experimental research. It was hoped that by doing so, the generalizability of findings to actual interpersonal relationships would be enhanced. In addition, it has been recognized in community psychology literature that empirical knowledge of social-psychological variables derived from laboratory studies may bear little to large resemblance to how these variables actually operate in more complex social settings. It was hoped that by utilizing the interactions of student and patient as the setting for research one could provide the context in which these variables derive their meaningfulness, a context which is often excluded or reproduced with shortcomings in the laboratory.

Consequently, the present study was also designed to examine the structure of "control" in the relationship and how it effects the cognitions and behaviors of the participants. Two types of structured control were examined. One was a relationship in which the members were mutually dependent on one another for achieving desired outcomes, and where each had some degree of control over the desired outcome of the other. This mutuality of control was called reciprocity. It was operationalized in the present study by having the patient determine the student's course grade. A second structure was a relationship in which only one member was dependent on the other for achieving a desired outcome and had little influence on the desired goal of the other. This structure was called nonreciprocity, and was operationalized by having the instructor determine the student's grade. In both conditions, the patient was considered dependent upon the student for assistance with the tasks of reintegration.

It was expected that this structural difference would result in a number of cognitive and behavioral changes on the part of both help-seeker and helper. One such change involved the self-perceptions of help-seekers. The role of help-seeker was thought to carry with it a view of oneself as helpless and dependent on others to provide solutions to one's own problems. Such a role may reinforce concepts of being incompetent to personally effect changes in a difficult situation. In a reciprocal relationship, the help-seeker is given an opportunity to control the desired outcome of the other person who is helping him, and as a result is likely to view himself as having some control over his own desired outcomes. To the extent the patient sees himself at release as competent to achieve his goals, he will be more likely to achieve a successful adaptation to community life. This line of reasoning led to the following hypotheses. *Hypothesis I:* Help seekers in a reciprocal relationship will have a more positive evaluation of themselves, and see themselves as more potent and effectual than persons in a nonreciprocal relationship. *Hypothesis II:* Patients in a reciprocal relationship with student companions will achieve higher levels of adaptation to community reintegration than persons in a nonreciprocal relationship.

A second set of outcomes involve the explanations the helper gives of the patient's behavior. Explanations of another's behavior can be grossly classified in terms of the cause specified for the behavior to be explained. The behavior may be viewed as being externally induced, *e.g.*, the result of external situational factors, or as internally caused, a product of motives or traits. Similarly, causal factors may be seen as temporary and immediate, *e.g.*, a function of the present circumstances, or enduring and permanent, *e.g.*, personality traits. Also, their impact on behavior may be viewed as relatively circumscribed or as broad and pervasive.

The explanations one uses to account for another person's behavior is likely to be affected by one's interactions with that person. As interactions progress between two people from a point of being strangers to one of knowing the other, their accounts of the other's behavior should change. Initial explanations should draw on stereotyped concepts determined by a small set of characteristics known about the person. For this reason, initial explanations are likely to emphasize internal, enduring, or dispositional causes of the other's behavior. As interaction and familiarity increase, recognition of the context in which behavior occurs is likely to also increase. Consequently a broader range of factors, including external and situational determinants would be considered in explaining the other's behavior. *Hypothesis III* follows from this discussion: Causal explanations of the other's behavior will reflect a shift from internal to external cuases with increasing familiarity in the relationship.

It is also likely that some explanations are more instrumental than others in arriving at a more positive, satisfying outcome. In a reciprocal relationship in which attainment of a desired outcome is determined by the behavior of both participants, it would be especially important to accurately account for the other's behavior in order to guage one's own complimentary response. Understanding of another's behavior may not have to be as accurate where one is not dependent on the other for a desired outcome. It could also be argued that understanding becomes more accurate when situational events are considered in addition to internal events. Consequently, *Hypothesis IV* was generated: Use of situational factors to explain the behavior of a partner will be greater for a person in a reciprocal relationship than one that is nonreciprocal.

It is also likely that reciprocity will influence the way members perceive one another. *Hypothesis V:* Persons in a reciprocal relationship will be more accurate in their perception of their partner than persons in a nonreciprocal relationship. To the extent situational explanations are communicated in the relationship, emphasis by *A* on external, situational causes of *B*'s behavior in addition to internal, dispositional causes is likely to result in *B* seeing *A* as more understanding and more similar to *B*. *Hypothesis VI:* Persons in a reciprocal relationship will perceive their partners as more accurately understanding, and more similar to themselves.

Reciprocity may also increase the degree of personal involvement and thereby raise the level of satisfaction of members in the relationship. *Hypothesis VII:* Persons in a reciprocal relationship will report a more satisfying experience than persons in a nonreciprocal relationship.

METHOD

Design

The design called for 18 selected college undergraduates who were assigned to one of 18 newly-released psychiatric patients as a student companion to assist in the transition from hospital to community. Dyads met for approximately eight weeks in the fall quarter, October to December, 1970. The student companion was instructed to utilize himself as a resource person in whatever ways possible to assist the patient in transition.

The role was not further specified for three reasons: First, the experience of project staff with patients after discharge was limited. It was not known what might be the typical needs of patients or ways of assisting that would be most helpful. Secondly, only two restrictions thought necessary for the combined welfare of patient and student were placed on referrals to the project (*i.e.*, no more than five years hospitalization and a diagnosis other than chronic psychiatric disorder). Thus a range of patient types were expected, suggesting a need for flexibility in response by the companion aide. The final consideration stemmed from faith in the natural human potential interested and bright young people could bring to a helping relationship.

Patients were randomly assigned to students, and pairs were randomly assigned to reciprocal or nonreciprocal treatments. At 4-week intervals during the relationship, the patient was interviewed and asked to describe his activities with the student. In the reciprocal relationship the patient was also asked for an evaluation of the student's performance in the helping role. Both patient and student were told that an evaluation would be made, that the evaluation would determine the student's course grade, and that the student would be informed of the evaluation in order to improve his performance in the relationship. In the nonreciprocal relationship, the patient was interviewed and asked only to describe their activities together. No evaluation was requested. Both patient and student in this group were informed that in no way was the interview to be used as an evaluation of the student's performance. They were also told that project staff, not the patient, would determine the student's grade in the course. Interviews were conducted by a patient hired as a research assistant specifically for this purpose and without participating in any of the experimental conditions.

Subjects

Patients. S_s were 18 male hospitalized psychiatric patients from a nearby VA Hospital (Brentwood). Patients with less than five years hospitalization, a diagnosis other than chronic psychiatric disorder, and who would stay in the area after discharge were eligible. Mean age for the sample was 35.3, mean hospital stay was less than 2 years, diagnosis was generally schizophrenia or alcoholism. Patients about to be released were referred at the discretion of the hospital staff and interviewed by a member of the research team. Participation in the project was voluntary.

Students. Student companions were 18 male college undergraduates who were enrolled in the project as a course for credit. Students were juniors or seniors with a major in psychology, and at least one completed course in related areas of abnormal psychology, personality, learning disorders, or exceptional children. Students were selected by the research staff on the basis of applications and personal interview. No one wishing to enroll was denied acceptance.

Procedure

Students and patients spent a minimum of 4 hours per week in face-to-face contact. Total length of contact ranged from 4 to 8 weeks with a mean of 6.3 weeks. Students provided transportation, accompanied the patient when he sought housing or employment, assisted in the completion of application forms, joined in recreational activities, visited in each other's homes, shared feelings and concerns, suggested a helpful perspective, and simply talked.

Students in each group met separately for an additional 2 hours per week with an advanced graduate student in clinical psychology to discuss theoretical and practical issues related to their contacts with patients. Discussion group leaders were uninformed of experimental conditions and hypotheses. Students were instructed not to discuss their experiences with students outside their group, and to direct their concerns about evaluation to the course instructor.

Measures

Four sets of measures were used.

1) *Semantic differentials.* Ratings of 20 polar adjectives to describe 7 concepts were obtained from patients and students using the semantic differential (S-D) adapted from Osgood, Suci, and Tannenbaum (1961). S-D ratings were made prior to initiating contacts between student and patient (Set 1), at the time of the patient's first interview (Set 2) and again at the conclusion of the project (Set 3). Concepts rated were: 1) mental hospital, 2) mental patient, 3) mental health worker, 4) college student, 5) myself, 6) my patient or my companion "I am about to meet" were added for Set 1 only], and 7) the way my patient (companion) sees himself. Concepts 1 thru 6 were rated at Set 1, 5-7 at Set 2, and 1 thru 7 at Set 3. In addition, students rated "my patient" at the end of each week of contact.

2) *Patient Interview Schedule.* Patient's description and evaluation of their companion and the project was recorded on a Patient Interview Schedule, consisting of 3 items asking for evaluation of program and student (*e.g.*, how satisfying do you feel the program has been thus far) and 17 items describing specific behaviors of their student (*e.g.*, talks about unimportant things). Each item was rated on a 9 point scale, "not at all" to "very much." An additional 9 items requested descriptive information about their activities with their companion.

3. *Relationship Inventory.* Patients and students also completed an 11-item Relationship Inventory at 4-week intervals during the project (Set 2 and 3). Items included such questions as "How much does the relationship satisfy your needs?" "How much do you both share in the planning of what you do?" Items were rated on a 7 point scale "not at all" to "very much." A total over all items provided an index of the extent of reciprocity achieved in the relationship.

4) *Daily logs.* The student kept a daily log in which he summarized his contacts with his patient, and reported in detail a discrete incident containing some specific behavior of the patient for each half-hour of contact. He then gave an account of the patient's behavior. These accounts were then analysed by independent raters to provide evidence of the causal factors used in the explanations by students.

5) *Follow-up data.* Information from hospital records as to status of the patient at 9-month follow-up (inpatient, outpatient, or discharged) and whether he had been readmitted since the project gave rather gross evidence of adjustment to community life.

Incomplete data

Patients were requested to return to the hospital twice during the project for an interview and to complete research scales. Patients were paid $2.50 per hour for each interview. Unfortunately this was insufficient inducement to some, despite extensive efforts to the contrary. The number of patients and students in each group completing the scales at each interview is listed in Table 1. Data obtained at the second interview (Set 3) are most incomplete, such that findings from these data should be considered only suggestive. Differences between the show and no show patients have not yet been determined.

TABLE 1

Number Persons Completing Research Scales at Each Interview.

	Intake (Set 1)	First Interview (Set 2)	Second Interview (Set 3)
Patients			
Reciprocal	8[1]	7	6[3]
Nonreciprocal	9	7	7
Students			
Reciprocal	9[1]	8	7[2]
Nonreciprocal	9	9	9

[1] Patient was reconsidered by hospital staff as inappropriate and subsequently dropped. Student data Set 1 retained.

[2] Student left University prior to completing last data set.

[3] S-D ratings on 2 of these Ss were incomplete.

RESULTS

Relationship Inventory

Total scores on the 11-item Relationship Inventory were combined for patients and students within treatments, for Set 2 and Set 3 data separately. The reciprocal group had higher scores for both data sets (56.21 and 55.92, respectively) compared to the nonreciprocal group, (53.44 and 52.94) reflecting greater reciprocity in the former as expected. However, the differences were not significant (ts < 1.0).

Hypothesis I

An analysis of the self-evaluations of patients from S-D ratings of the concept "myself," using Set 2 and Set 3 data was not complete at the time of this report. However, an analysis of ratings for "myself" and for "the person I am about to meet" was performed for Set 1 ratings. These ratings were made before the first contact between patient and student, and before the effect of the treatments was experienced. Consequently, treatment groups were combined and the significance of the difference between means for students versus patients was obtained for each adjective using t tests for independent samples.

Of the 40 possible comparisons, 22 were significantly different at the .05 level or beyond (two-tailed probabilities), a number well beyond the two comparisons that could be expected to be significant by chance factors alone given this many comparisons. The adjectives for which significant differences were obtained are given in Table 2. With the exception of "hard-soft" ratings, patients rated themselves significantly more negative than did students. In contrast, patients rated their student companion more favorably on 11 adjectives than students rated their patient partner.

The perceptions of self and expectations of other characterizing each group could certainly be expected to have an impact on their initial interaction. To the extent patient evaluations of self would become more positive over the course of contacts, Hypothesis I would suggest the increase would be greater for persons in the reciprocal relationships.

TABLE 2

Differences in Set 1 S-D Ratings for Students and Patients,

Treatments Combined

	Students	Patients	t	p value
Concept: <u>myself</u>				
true-false	2.00	3.12	2.43	.021
wise-foolish	2.82	4.12	2.33	.027
sweet-sour	3.06	4.65	2.75	.010
strong-weak	2.94	4.56	2.47	.019
hard-soft	5.24	4.06	2.09	.044
sharp-dull	1.76	3.29	3.24	.003
safe-dangerous	2.18	3.82	2.53	.016
good-bad	1.88	2.82	2.11	.043
pleasant-unpleasant	1.71	3.00	2.77	.009
helpful-harmful	1.47	2.65	2.20	.036
relaxed-tense	5.59	7.53	2.85	.008
Concept: <u>my companion</u>				
wise-foolish	3.59	1.76	4.69	.001
fair-unfair	3.59	2.18	3.75	.001
strong-weak	4.88	2.53	5.01	.001
rugged-delicate	5.06	3.47	3.10	.004
sharp-dull	4.41	2.12	5.85	.001
warm-cold	4.06	2.41	3.80	.001
active passive	4.59	2.24	4.31	.001
fast-slow	4.65	2.76	3.91	.001
helpful-harmful	2.65	1.71	2.54	.016
relaxed-tense	7.41	3.82	6.68	.001
friendly-unfriendly	4.18	2.82	2.51	.017

Hypothesis II

Follow-up data for patients in the two treatment groups
are given in Table 3, along with those for a group of "no-treat-
ment" patients having no companion at transition. Persons in
this group were patients referred to the project but who did

TABLE 3

Hospital Status at 9 Months after Project Ended

Group	No. pts.	No. pts. available at follow-up	No. pts. readmitted since project	No. pts. not readmitted	Proportion not readmitted
Reciprocal	8	7	4	3	.43
Nonreciprocal	9	9	4	5	.55
Non-participants	6	6	4	2	.33

Group	No. pts.	No. pts. available at follow-up	Status of pt. at follow-up Inpatient	Outpatient	Discharged	Proportion Outpatient or Discharged
Reciprocal	8	7	2	2	3	.71
Nonreciprocal	9	9	0	7	2	1.00
Non-participants	6	6	2	2	2	.66

not participate, either out of disinterest or because they were likely not to remain in the area.

The two treatment groups had a somewhat larger proportion of patients who stayed out of the hospital during the 9-month interval or who were on outpatient or discharge status at follow-up. The numbers are small and the differences between groups are certainly not substantial. Yet, these gross indicators of community adjustment lend some support to the effectiveness of student companions at release. The figures also suggest patients in the nonreciprocal group had "better adjustment" than patients in the reciprocal group. These findings are contrary to expectations for the therapeutic value of a reciprocal relationship.

Hypotheses III and IV

Daily logs of students are presently being analyzed for use of situational explanations in accounting for patient behavior. These findings will be presented in a later report (Blechman and Freitag, in preparation).

Hypothesis V

Accuracy in perceiving one's partner was obtained by correlating student and patient S-D ratings of the way their partner sees himself (concept 7) with their partner's S-D rating of self (concept 5) for Set 2 data only. Set 3 data were excluded since these ratings were available for less than half the pairs in the reciprocal treatment. Product moment correlations for patients and students combined was .454 for the reciprocal group and .495 for the nonreciprocal group. The difference was not significant, thereby giving no support to Hypothesis V.

Hypotheses VI and VII

Patient responses to the 20 items of the Patient Interview Schedule were intercorrelated for Set 2 data only. These correlations are shown in Table 4. Items which correlated significantly ($r \geq .66$, $p < .05$) were thought to share some meaning for the patient. Three clusters of items with correlations of .66 or better were obtained. The first cluster involved items 1, 2, 3, 5, and 9 and seemed to represent a "general level of satis-

TABLE 4

Product Moment Correlations for Items of Patient Interview Schedule, Set 2, Patients Combined.

Item	1	2	3	4	5	6	7	8	9	10	11	 17
1. getting what I expected												
2. satisfied with the program	.76**											
3. helpful	.73**	.97**										
4. keeps appointments												
5. arrives on time	.77**											
6. calls ahead if late or to cancel				.66*								
7. appears neat & clean												
8. interested in what I say												
9. asks too many questions	-.70**				-.67*		-.91**					
10. asks embarrassing questions												
11. talks about unimportant things												
12. talks about self												
13. gives advice												
14. says things I don't understand							-.95**					
15. seems nervous									.86**			
16. makes me feel comfortable									.66*		.79**	
17. have some things in common						.68**						
18. have similar experiences												
19. seems concerned about me						.92**						
20. seems to understand how I feel						.71**						.66*

* p < .02
** p < .01

faction" with student companion. The second was a grouping of
items 9, 14, 15, and 11, describing a kind of "nervous questioning." This cluster was negatively correlated with items 1 and 5
of the first cluster. Two of the highest negative correlations
were also obtained for items 9 and 14 of this second cluster,
and item 7, "appears neat and clean." A third set of intercor-
relations for items 6, 17, 19 and 20 reflect a "similarity, regard, and understanding" cluster.

Mean group ratings for each item were obtained and compared,
using t tests for independent samples. Only one difference was
significant. Patients in the reciprocal group reported their
students asked more embarassing or difficult to answer questions
(t=2.17, p   .05 two-tailed), a significance to be expected by
chance given the number of comparisons made. Consequently, the
data do not support either hypothesis. However, the direction
of the differences was as predicted. Patients in the reciprocal
treatment had higher ratings for items 6, 17, 19 and 20, the
"similarity, regard, understanding" cluster, consistent with
Hypothesis VI. Similarly, reciprocal patients had higher scores
on 4 of the 5 items making up the "general level of satisfaction"
cluster as stated in Hypothesis VII.

DISCUSSION AND CONCLUSIONS

The central aim of this project was met in providing the
ex-mental patient with assistance in handling the tasks that
accompany transition from hospital to community life. The critical question of how effective was the companion in facilitating
successful adaptation to the community was answered only indirectly by the patient's hospital status during the 9 months following termination of the project. Having a student companion
at release improved but did not demonstrably alter the tendency
for these patients to return to the hospital. However, the esti-
mates of adjustment were gross ones. A more reliable index such
as the Community Adaptation Scale (Roen, Ottenstein, Rosenblum,
Cooper and Burnes, 1966) would clarify the program's effectiveness for patient adjustment. Patients' evaluations of the student as helper were generally favorable, suggesting that from the
patient's perspective, there was something gained in having a
student companion at release. Further experimentation of student
companion aides seems warranted.

To the extent the student was helpful, the patient had either not been rehospitalized or was on outpatient or discharge
status 9 months after the project ended. The percentage of patients in these two outcomes was greater for persons in the non-

reciprocal condition compared to the reciprocal group, contrary to expectations. If reliable, the differences imply that being in a reciprocal relationship and having to evaluate one's helper for a grade may have tended to hamper, rather than facilitate, community adjustment.

The basic premise underlying this study was that the problems at hospital release were problems of transition in social roles. A further direction for research in this area would be to identify the characteristics of each role and the point at which transition becomes hazardous for the individual. Intervention might involve a more dynamic approach to crisis resolution with individuals or a restructuring of the social roles. By approaching the situation as a problem in social roles, and working forward in time, intervention could become one of tertiary prevention (Caplan, 1964). The aim would be to reduce the incidence of hazard and the likelihood of rehospitalization for all individuals.

The tasks of community adjustment are likely not to be the same for all psychiatric patients upon hospital release. A direction for further examination would be to accompany a particular group of hospitalized patients, *e.g.*, the neuropsychiatric casualties returning from the Vietnam War, and identify the specific tasks and processes of community adjustment experienced by them at transition.

The project was also successful in creating a new helping role for the college undergraduate. It was surprising, and somewhat frightening at times, to see how important the students became for some patients. One patient after being gone from his apartment for several days with his whereabouts unknown to his landlady and social worker, called his student companion from out of town to say he was alright. Another instance of closeness was reflected in the difficulty both participants had in terminating the relationship after only 8 weeks of contact. At the same time it was gratifying to see the sensitivity and skill some students demonstrated in handling the momentary crises of helping seriously disturbed persons. The experience of the authors strengthens the belief that the role of companion aide, while a demanding one, can be carried out effectively by a nonprofessional.

The dependency of some patients on the student as his only means of social contact suggests that in replication of the project, the dyad work toward developing other sources of social contact for the patient. Activities with other persons could foster additional friendships and provide useful continuity for the patient when the project relationships terminate officially. It may be instrumental in this regard to utilize other patients in the role of companion aide.

The obtained relationship between student's nervous questioning and patient's negative appraisal of his helpfulness and his physical appearance suggests that certain behaviors of the helper emitted early in the contacts may be perceived by the patient as noxious. The nontherapeutic value of direct questioning has been mentioned elsewhere (Goodman, 1970), but had not previously been shown to be related to an evaluative judgment of the therapist by the patient. It is interesting that such a judgement was expressed toward the physical attributes of the person which have no apparent relationship to therapeutic skills. The finding suggests an interesting hypothesis for further investigation, namely that liking of the therapist is a function of certain specific response modes of the therapist, in addition to certain qualities the therapist possesses. The finding further supports the notion that the student-patient relationship is an appropriate place in which to examine certain social-psychological variables like interpersonal attraction.

The interrelatedness of ratings of similarity with perceived concern and understanding is consistent with the psychotherapy literature showing that perceived similarity is related to perceived conditions of accurate empathy, regard, and genuineness of the therapist (Truax and Carkhuff, 1967; Carkhuff and Pierce, 1967). The surprising thing is that this relationship was found with college undergraduates and VA patients who are objectively dissimilar in several respects, *e.g.*, age, educational level, marital status, military experience, political and social ideologies, and dress (about a third of the students had long hair). Patients mean ratings on the similarity items (*i.e.*, have some things in common, have similar experiences as you) were at midpoint or below, suggesting perceived similarity was not high. Consequently, a student companion program that maximized perceived similarity by selecting patients of similar age, etc. would appear to enhance the likelihood of therapeutic benefits for the patient.

Use of the helping relationship as an opportunity for research was less rewarding. Of the four hypotheses concerning reciprocity for which data were available at the time of this report, none were supported. The failure to find significant effects of reciprocity may reflect a failure to adequately create the desired experimental conditions. It should be noted that mean patients' ratings on the Patient Interview Schedule revealed a generally higher score on each item, regardless of content, for patients in the reciprocal group. This could represent a response bias favoring an inflated (although not necessarily favorable) rating for students in this group. It appears patients took their grading role seriously. However, there were no significant differences between the two treatment groups on the Relationship Inventory, a measure designed to tap degree of reciprocity. Whatever the effect of the manipulation, it was neither strong nor certain to equalize control among the participants.

Despite the discouraging results, the use of the non-professional helping relationship as the setting for empirical research seems warranted. The non-professional status of the relationship, while precluding research on certain questions of psychotherapy (*e.g.*, comparative effectiveness of therapeutic methodologies) may actually be ideal to examine more discrete variables thought to relate to therapeutic effectiveness, *e.g.* the impact on the patient of asking too many questions too early, or the manner in which they are asked. These more discrete variables may be more easily isolated in a non-professional relationship where their effects are not confounded by other variables of level of therapist experience, theoretical orientation, and training.

College students have not been viewed as the vehicles for empirical research in the way suggested here. Their helping relationships with patients have not been explored as a legitimate context in which to examine social-psychological variables. The experience of this project suggests that college students can be effective instruments in creating structured social interactions as well as providing data on their own experiences as participants.

The model appears fruitful in a variety of ways. It has the combined advantages of a teaching device which places students in an activity in which they can test out and develop their own interpersonal skills, explore individual behavior in community settings, and acquire research skills within the context of empirical investigation. It has the additional advantage of providing faculty the manpower for conducting experimental research with clinically-related problems in community settings. The project is currently the model for an undergraduate field laboratory in clinical and community psychology at UCLA.

NOTE: - This research was supported by UCLA Academic Senate Research Grant No. 2505. The authors wish to thank the staff and residents of the Brentwood Hospital, Veterans Administration Center, Los Angeles for their cooperation and participation in this project.

REFERENCES

Camp, R. P. and Onnenebo, F. Discharged psychiatric patients visits to a former treatment center: A nursing dilemma. *Journal of Psychiatric Nursing & Mental Health Services,* 1968, *6* (4), 213-218.

Caplan, G. *Principles of preventive psychiatry.* New York: Basic Books Inc., 1964.

Carkhuff, R. R. and Pierce, R. Differential effects of therapist race and social class upon patient depth of self-exploration in the initial clinical interview. *Journal of Consulting Psychology,* 1967, *31,* 632-634.

Cowen, E., Zax, M., and Laird, J. A college student volunteer program in the elementary school setting. *Community Mental Health,* 1966, *2,* 319-328.

Freeman, H. E., and Simmons, D. G. *The mental patient comes home.* New York: Wiley, 1963.

Goodman, G. Companionship as therapy: The use of non-professional talent. In Hart, J. T., and Tomlinson, T. M. (Eds.), *New directions in client centered therapy.* New York: Houghton Mifflin Co., 1970, 348-381.

Greenblatt, M., Levinson, D. J., Klerman, G. L. (Eds.), *Mental patients in transition.* Springfield, Illinois: Chas. Thomas, 1961.

Guerney, B. G. *Psychotherapeutic agents: New roles for professionals, parents, and teachers.* New York: Holt, Rinehart, and Winston, 1969.

Holzberg, J. D., Knapp, R. H., and Turner, J. L. College students as companions to the mentally ill. In E. A. Cowen, E. A. Gardener, and M. Zax (Eds.), *Emergent approaches to mental health problems.* New York: Appleton-Century-Crofts, 1967.

Klein, D., and Lindemann, E. Preventive intervention in individual and family crisis situations. In G. Caplan (ed.), *Prevention of mental disorders in children.* New York: Basic Books, 1961, 283-306.

Levinson, D. J. and Gallagher, E. B. *Patienthood in the mental hospital.* Boston: Houghton Mifflin Co., 1964.

Newton, M. R., and Brown, R. D.   A preventive approach to developmental problems in school children.   In Bower and Hollister (Eds.), *Behavioral science frontiers in education*. New York: J. Wiley, 1967.

Osgood, C. E., Suci, G., and Tannenbaum, P. H.   *The measurement of meaning*.   Urbana, Illinois: University of Illinois Press, 1961.

Purvis, S. A., and Miekunins, R. W.   Effects of the community follow-up on post hospitilization adjustment of psychiatric patients. *Community Mental Health Journal*, 1970, *6* (5) 374-382.

Roen, S. R., Ottenstein, D., Rosenblum, G., Cooper, S. and Burnes, A. J.   *Communication patterns in community aftercare*.   Quincy, Massachusetts: Southern Shore Mental Health Center, 1966.

Sarbin, T. R.   A role-theory perspective for community psychology: The structure of social identity.   In D. Adelson and B. L. Kalis (Eds.), *Community psychology and mental health*. Scranton, Pennsylvania: Chandler Publishing Co., 1970, 89-113.

Stewart, A., Selkirk, S., & Sydiaha, D.   Patterns of adjustment of discharged psychiatric patients as measured by mailed questionnaires. *Community Mental Health Journal*, 1969, *5*, 314-319.

Truax, C. B., and Carkhuff, R. R.   *Toward effective counseling and psychotherapy*.   Chicago: Aldine Publishing Co., 1967.

Umbarger, C. C., Morrison, A. P., Dalsimer, J. S. and Breggin, P. R.   *College students in a mental hospital*.   New York: Grune and Stratton, 1962.

10: MANAGEMENT OF THE BEREAVEMENT CRISIS

This chapter by Jon Williams deals with the theory and application of crisis intervention for the bereaved. Williams begins by reviewing the thinking of others on the phenomena associated with the loss of a loved one. He continues by elaborating his own model of mourning and grief, which has its roots in Gestalt psychology and psychodrama theory. The author distinguishes between normal and pathological reactions to death; he proposes that crisis intervention may lessen the frequency with which pathological reactions occur.

The action program described by Williams involve consultation and training of clergy. Recognizing that the clergyman is often a primary resource for the bereaved, Williams sought to strengthen this "natural mental health service delivery system" as Levy in an earlier chapter labeled such resources. In cooperation with a clerical association, Williams recruited a group of clergymen of various faiths for the program. This group met with the author over a period of eight months of weekly sessions. The training procedure included the assignment of relevant readings, the presentation of a guide for clerical efforts, and the opportunity for consultative discussion sessions on a group or individual basis. Discussions were centered on actual contacts with the bereaved as they were encountered by the clerical trainees. An effort was made to assess the impact of the consultation upon the clergymen; findings suggested that the program had been effective in altering churchmen's conceptions and strategies for handling the crisis of bereavement.

Two features of William's project are particularly notable. First, as has already been commented, the program did not aim at creating a new service group; rather, it was designed to improve the functioning of a group already being utilized by members of the community. Second, as discussed in Freitag's chapter, it was assumed *a priori* that an identifiable event, hospital release for Freitag and the death of a loved one for Williams, would be generally associated with a period of crisis. Operating upon this assumption it was possible for Williams, as for

Freitag, to work toward training or providing help-givers to aid in the management of crisis before it could have lastingly destructive consequences.

CRISIS INTERVENTION AMONG THE BEREAVED:

A MENTAL HEALTH CONSULTATION PROGRAM FOR CLERGY

Jon E. Williams

Bereavement as the complex response to loss of a significant object has recently become a topic of major interest among mental-health workers. Averill (1968) has delineated *mourning* and *grief* as the two major components of bereavement and has suggested that both function to maintain social cohesiveness and stability.

Popular articles and books (Liebermann, 1970; Mitford, 1963; Woodward, 1970) have made dramatic appeals for rescuing and revitalizing mourning rituals and rites in a culture in which death is considered "UnAmerican." Mourning rituals and rites are important to community psychology because they provide the socio-cultural supports which help to determine the negative or positive consequences of bereavement.

The importance of grief has been suggested by Knight, a psychiatrist, (Jackson, 1963) who believes grief to be *the* phenomenon around which modern psychosomatic medicine revolves and by Parkes, a British psychiatrist, (1965) who holds grief to be *the* key to understanding psychopathology. As Parkes states it, "grief may prove to be as important to psychopathology as inflamation is to pathology."

The present paper defines bereavement within the framework of crisis theory, establishes a need for crisis intervention in both the mourning and grief aspects of bereavement, and provides a description and an evaluation of a consultation with a group of clergymen concerned with crisis intervention among the bereaved.

CRISIS THEORY AS FRAMEWORK FOR STUDY OF BEREAVEMENT

Bereavement, when defined within the framework of crisis

140

theory, not only invites a broad interdisciplinary perspective in determining what the problem is but also helps to focus the practical issues of constructive intervention in determining what to do about the problem.

Modern crisis theory has its roots in a now classic study of bereavement by Lindemann (1944). The concept of crisis, as formulated by Lindemann (1944) and later restated by Caplan (1964), refers to the state of the reacting individual and/or group at a *turning point* in a hazardous situation which threatens integrity or wholeness. Paraphrasing Thomas (Volkart, 1951), the state of crisis serves as a catalyst that disturbs old habits, evokes new responses, and becomes a major factor in chartering new developments, the outcomes of which may be either positive or negative. Thus, bereavement may be defined as a crisis or transition period the adaptive function of which is individual and social integration.

Mourning and Grief: A Social, Psychological, and Physiological Adaptation to Loss

Mourning and grief, as interrelated components of bereavement, are the processes through which the bereaved achieve social, psychological, and physiological adaptation to the loss of a significant object.

Mourning represents conventional behavior determined by the mores, beliefs, and customs of society whereas grief comprises a stereotyped set of psychological and physiological reactions of probable biological origins (Averill, 1968). Although these response patterns may occur independently of each other, they usually are closely related and may even complement one another.

Mourning rites and rituals generally serve two purposes: they help reinforce the religious and social structure of the group and thereby maintain group solidarity and cohesion, and, when no conflict between the society and the individual is involved, they help assuage the emotions of the bereaved and thereby provide a supportive social context within which grief work seeks resolution. Rituals and rites connected with death are almost always of a religious nature, the function of which, is to work against destructive fantasy and illusion and toward a framework of reality.

Among the more useful concepts for understanding the interrelatedness of both the group and the individual and mourning and grief in bereavement are the concepts of the "social atom"

taken from psychodrama (Moreno, 1947) and of "closure" taken
from Gestalt psychology.

The "social atom" is the smallest social unit which includes both the individual and the people (near and distant) to
whom the individual is emotionally related at any given time.
Bereavement necessitates a social psychological readjustment of
those who remain in the "atom" after a significant member dies.
Without adequate cultural supports in the form of mourning rituals and rites, the "social atom" may disintegrate. In America
the primary social atom is the nuclear family. A death in the
family, as Hinton (1967) has noted, all too often begins a series of schisms which ultimately destroys family solidarity and
cohesion. Family therapists (e.g., Jensen and Wallace, 1967;
Paul and Grosser, 1965) are increasingly advocating crisis intervention to avert the destruction of schisms in bereaved families.

Gestalt theory suggests that man must bring about closure
in all of his experiences; that all of an individual's or group's
experiences must be interrelated; and that all individuals and
groups struggle to achieve such closure. Mourning and grief
taken separately and together, appear to be attempts to bring
about closure. That is, all interpersonal and social relationships may be conceived of as some form of closure. At the time
of death the closure is broken and the social ties are threatened with further breaks. Diagrammatically, there is a gap in
the circle of the surviving individual and "social atom." In
a sense, the bereavement crisis is a response to threat of sepa-
ration and isolation which calls for new closure following the
loss of a prior relationship. At the time of loss, then, both
mourning and grief attempt to heal the break in the existential
continuum and thereby achieve new wholeness.

Unfortunately, there is growing evidence to suggest a dis-
solution and breakdown of Anglo-American cultural supports for
the bereaved (Gorer, 1965; Lieberman, 1970; Marris, 1958;
Parkes, 1965; Woodward, 1970). One of the more balanced statements of the cultural problem is that of Mandelbaum (1959):

> American culture has, in certain respects,
> and for some Americans, become deritualized.
> Persons bereaved by death sometimes find
> that they have no clear prescription as to
> what to do next. In such cases each has to
> work out a solution for himself. After the
> typical period of shock and disorganization,
> these mourners can receive little help towards
> personal reorganization.

Summarizing a review of attitudinal research, Gerber (1969) has suggested that the prevailing public attitude toward death and its consequences is a combination of evasion, euphemism, and stoical acceptance. The dominant attitude, however, is one of denial. As Feifel (1959) and others (Fulton, 1965; Gorer, 1965; Lieberman, 1970) have suggested, death and its consequences have fast become *the* taboo in modern Anglo-American culture. Unless we can revitalize our mourning rituals and rites, Americans will continue to have ever greater difficulty in attaining a positive resolution of the bereavement crisis.

Together with mourning, grief as the second component of the bereavement crisis also serves an adaptive function on behalf of individual and social integration. Unlike mourning, grief is primarily a psycho-physiological or psycho-somatic phenomenon, probably of biological origins (Averill, 1968; Volkan, 1966).

Unfortunately, the quality and extent of investigation into both the physiological and psychological aspects of grief leave much to be desired. Beginning with Freud (1917), most of the psychoanalytic work on grief has been theoretical and used merely to illustrate other analytic concepts and concerns (Siggin, 1966). The work of grief, according to Freud (1917), is the difficult, timely, and painful task of "decathecting" libido from a lost object and reinvesting it in the new reality situation. Although far from sufficient, the work of Freud and his followers has illuminated both intrapsychic and interpersonal meanings of grief and has recognized that grief is not in itself pathological, thereby suggesting a so-called "normal" grief reaction from which "pathological" variations diverge.

In the first semi-empirical work on bereavement, Lindemann (1944) demonstrated the difference between normal and pathological grief reactions. Based on the work of Lindemann (1944) and his followers (Averill, 1968; Baler & Golde, 1964; Bowlby, 1960, 1961, 1963; Clayton *et al.*, 1967; Marris, 1958; Parkes, 1964, 1965, 1967; Volkan, 1966), the ensuing is an explication of normal grief as set within the context of crisis theory and presented without due regard for significant individual and situational differences.

Normal Grief Reactions. Normal grief, like other crises, is a time of intense mental anguish and of reduced psychological and physiological resistance to stress with little past history of experience to draw upon for support. In the normal grief process the bereaved pass through three stages: shock, despair, or disorganization and recovery or reorganization. The outcome of normal grief is a positive reorganization in which the bereaved are reunited with the living community and gain a new symbolic identification with those who have died.

The "shock" stage of grief frequently begins with a phase of "numbing" which may last from a few days to about a week, is sometimes interrupted with outbursts of intense anger and/or distress, and is usually accompanied by physiological changes similar to those observed in other periods of acute stress. The shock stage usually ends after a few weeks of on-and-off yearning and searching for the return of the dead person. This final phase of stage one is frequently characterized by denial and disbelief.

As the reality of loss prevails against denial and disbelief, a second stage of "despair" and "disorganization" ensues. This is a period of intense mental anguish interrupted with brief stretches of relative homeostasis and psychological equilibrium. It usually lasts from several weeks to several months. The second stage is characterized by apathy, withdrawal, brief periods of disorganized overactivity; by preoccupation with thoughts of the deceased; by difficulty in concentrating on routine tasks or in initiating new activities; by a variety of psychosomatic complaints including gastrointestinal problems, sleep disturbance, weight loss, and excessive fatigue; by a mixture of feelings including anxiety, hostility, guilt, helplessness, and despair; and by an unusually persistent depression which is unalleviated by rest and associated with a deficiency in central noradrenergic mechanisms. The depression of grief, according to Davis (1964), is based upon the extinction of behavior formerly directed toward the lost object. The extinction of such behaviors is a necessary precondition to the third stage of recovery and reorganization.

The final stage of normal grief marks the beginning of recovery and reorganization and includes adaptation and adjustment to the reality of loss and establishment of new relationships and attachments which enhance group cohesiveness and solidarity. Among the gains of the recovery period is the realization of ability to cope successfully with loss resulting from death and to reinvest oneself in those who remain. Those who fail to adequately recover from loss vary away from the norm into what have been called "pathological grief reactions."

Pathological Grief Reactions. In addition to the increased probability of the early death of those who grieve unsuccessfully (Kraus & Lilienfeld, 1959; Ress & Lutkins, 1967; Young *et al.*, 1963), it is not at all unusual to trace the beginning of neuroses, psychoses, and psychosomatic disorders to unresolved or pathological grief. What may have begun as a process of normal grief may end in morbidity or maladjustment.

According to Lindemann (1944) and Parkes (1965), grief may be regarded as pathological if any of the symptoms of normal grief are unduly delayed, prolonged, or inhibited, or if the process of grief is excessively intensive or exaggerated.

The persistent absence of any emotion may signal undue delay in the beginning of the work of grief and lead to pathology. Deutsch (1937), for example, suggested that grief can never be successfully denied and will manifest itself in psychiatric conditions such as periodic depressions if not manifested openly. Lindemann (1944) found that some of his bereaved patients were preoccupied with grief about a person who died many years ago. He indicated that undue delay, consisting of displacement or absence of affect, may sometimes be owing to a negative neurotic identification with the dead person such that the bereaved "lives as if he were dead."

Prolongation of grief may be due to a delay in beginning the process, or to a retarding of the process once it has begun, or both. Since such is a matter of degree the dividing line is often unclear. Prolongation, like the absence of grief, provides an avenue of avoiding the anxiety associated with the difficult and unpleasant tasks involved in grief; such avoidance of anxiety is frequently the basis of a variety of pathologies. Seeking to avoid the pain of grief, the bereaved often deny the reality of their loss. Fleming and Altschul (1963) have reported cases in which the patients suffered the loss of parents in adolescence but had never grieved and continued covertly to deny the reality of the loss. Denial of real loss, according to Jackson (1957), may take at least two pathological forms: over-idealizing the lost object so that unpleasant features of the relationship remain unprocessed, and acting out of denial in promiscuity or dissipation.

Related to both delay and prolongation of grief is what Averill (1968) has labelled "inhibited grief" which is defined as "a lasting inhibition of many of the manifestations of normal grief, but with the appearance of other symptoms, for instance, somatic complaints, in their stead." Inhibition of grief is commonly found among children (Rochlin, 1965), adolescents (Shoor & Speed, 1963), and the elderly (Stern *et al.*, 1951).

Another group of pathological grief reactions is that which Lindemann (1944) called "distortion" or "grief reactions of abnormal intensity." Any one of the symptoms of normal grief may be exaggerated out of all proportion. Such exaggeration usually represents a conflict with the lost person. These intensified or exaggerated reactions are themselves pathological, but they may in addition cause an abnormal prolongation of the grief

process. Lindemann (1944) listed the following distortions:
guilt with an obvious need for punishment; somatic symptoms
such as insomnia, anorexia, or diarrhea; acquisition of symptoms belonging to the last illness of the deceased; denial of
feelings and an appearance of woodenness; altered relationships
to friends; and furious hostility and irritability in relationship to specific persons.

Related to and considered by some to be inseparable from
pathological grief reactions are those psychiatric and somatic
illnesses precipitated by bereavement. Examples of psychiatric
disorders are anxiety states, phobic conditions, hysteria, obsessional reactions, and manic-depression states including agi-
tated depression, anergic depression, and hypomania (Anderson,
1949; Barnacle, 1949; Lehrman, 1956; MacCurdy, 1925; Peck, 1939;
Roth, 1959). Among the somatic illnesses thought to be sometimes precipitated by bereavement are ulcerative colitis and
rheumatoid arthritis (Lindemann, 1950), asthma (McDermott &
Cobb, 1939); leukemia (Greene & Miller, 1958), hyperthyroidism
(Lidz, 1949), and osteoarthritis (Parkes, 1964).

Pathological grief or "the refusal to mourn" interferes
with the process of "keeping current" or living in the "now."
Its consequences are disruption, disorganization, disintegration,
and both intrapsychic and interpersonal conflict. A systematic
program of crisis intervention among the bereaved is needed not
only to prevent or decrease the negative consequences of the
higher incidence of morbidity, maladjustment, and mortality
among those who are grieving but also to assuage the necessary
pain of grief and enhance the growth and development that can
come through successful coping with crises.

CRISIS INTERVENTION: TAKING CARE OF THE BEREAVED

Crisis intervention has been defined by Parad (1965) as the
process of "entering into the life situation of an individual,
family, or group to alleviate the impact of a crisis-inducing
stress in order to help mobilize the resources of those directly
affected, as well as those who are in the significant 'social
orbit.'"

The most appropriate persons for entering into the life
situation of the bereaved are the clergy, not only because they
are charged with developing and administering funeral rites and
rituals on behalf of the individual and community but also because they are the caretakers closest and with most natural
entre to those whom Sudnow (1967) has referred to as the

"legitimately bereaved." The clergyman is least likely to be rejected by the bereaved because of the congruence of the needs of the bereaved at the time of loss and the functions assigned to the clergy on behalf of the bereaved and because the clergyman is the caretaker most likely to have been consulted before in times of trouble (Gurin *et al.*, 1960).

A MENTAL HEALTH CONSULTATION PROGRAM FOR CLERGY

Recognizing bereavement as a crisis threatening the wholeness of both individuals and the community and accepting the clergy as the most appropriate caretaker of the bereaved, a mental health consultation program was designed for the training and support of clergy in crisis intervention among the bereaved. The program was a joint effort between the author, who was at that time assigned to the Southwest Team of the Area C Community Mental Health Center in Washington, D.C., and the Clergy Association of Southwest Washington.

The primary purposes of the consultation were fourfold: to provide specialized training in crisis counseling and intervention among the bereaved, to teach group process as a means of experiential continuing education among the clergy, to establish a closer communication link between the Community Mental Health Center and the clergy-caretakers, and to assess clergy attitudes toward the bereaved and evaluate effects of consultation on these attitudes.

After several weeks of meetings between the author and members of the clergy association the consultation began with a total of eleven clergy participants representing Protestant, Catholic, and Jewish traditions. Two of the eleven were "clergy-interns" still in training; the remaining nine represented different congregations. One of the clergy-interns dropped out after the second session because of illness. The rest of the group met with the consultant for weekly two hour sessions over a period of eight months, two months beyond an original six month contract.

At the suggestion of the consultant, the group agreed to spend the first six weeks responding to a series of papers read prior to each session which covered the following topics: Bereavement; Mourning and Grief; Grief: Normal and Pathological; Healing Aspects of Funeral and Religious Practices; The Shiva as a Therapeutic Model; Tactical Guidelines for Crisis Intervention Among the Bereaved; and Ministering to the Bereaved Family; Facilitating Adaptive Family Interaction Patterns Resulting from

Loss of a Family Member.

During the initial six weeks each participant adopted at
least one bereaved individual or family to follow through the
bereavement crisis for at least six months. In addition to bereaved "parishioners", several of the clergy also adopted
"unchurched" bereaved persons referred to the consultation by
the public health nurses in Southwest Washington.

After the initial discussion sessions, the participants
presented for group supervision and consultation situations and
problems encountered among the bereaved. Individual sessions
with the consultant were available upon request. Both individual and group sessions were used primarily for "client-centered"
and "consultee-centered" consultation (Caplan, 1964). Some
attention was also given to what Caplan (1964) has called "pro-
gram-centered administrative consultation" focused on two concerns: (a) the development of "lay support" or "widowed-to-
widowed" groups (Silverman, 1967) and (b) the development of
programs for the "re-examination and revitalization" of traditional funeral rites and rituals (Irion, 1954; Jackson, 1963;
Kidorf, 1963, 1966). Several special sessions were concerned
with "preventive opportunities in childhood bereavement" after
it became evident that the bereavement process among children
was poorly understood and frequently given little attention or
ignored.

Although each participant developed his own style of intervention, the following is a description of the tactical methods
adapted from Gerber (1969) for guiding the consultees in crisis
intervention among the bereaved:

1. Permitting and guiding the bereaved to put into words
   and express the affects involved in:
   (a) the pain, sorrow and finality of bereavement;
   (b) a review of the relationship to the deceased;
   (c) feeling of love, guilt, and hostility toward
       the deceased.

2. Acquainting the bereaved with the existence and/or
   understanding of alterations in his emotional reactions.

3. Assisting the bereaved to find an acceptable formulation of his future relationship to the psychic re-
   presentation of the deceased.

4. Acting as a "primer and/or programmer" of some of the
   activities of the bereaved and organizing among available, suitable friends or relatives a flexible, modest
   scheme for the same purpose.

5. Assisting the bereaved in dealing with reality sit-
    uations, care of children, legal problems, etc.

6. Mediating referrals to family physician for prescrip-
    tions of psychic energizers, tranquilizers and hypnot-
    ics if necessary for excessive depression, anxiety,
    and insomnia.

7. The offer of assistance in making future plans.

8. As a rule the following is to be avoided:
    (a) Interpretation of key defenses and highly
        charged warded-off, unconscious trends.
    (b) Excessive solicitude and overprotection of
        the bereaved.

9. The baseline attitude of the caretaker, from which
    appropriate departures may be made, is to be one of
    compassionate but temperate concern, avoiding senti-
    mentality and over-identification. The caretaker
    should recognize the full extent of the emotional
    loss but gently convey to the bereaved -- after the
    subsidence of the acute, initial, intense phase of
    grief -- that it is the normal, expected course that
    he recover like anyone else and that the bereaved
    person does indeed possess the required inner strength
    for this.

10. Special emphasis is placed on a "family-systems"
    approach to bereavement, on recognizing the interper-
    sonal as well as the intrapsychic aspects of bereave-
    ment. If possible the bereaved are to be seen in
    their homes. They are encouraged to discuss in a
    family gathering their separate feelings not only
    about the deceased but also about each other. As
    a family group they are guided toward a new social
    arrangement which incorporates the roles and tasks
    once fulfilled by the deceased.

EVALUATION

During the eight months of the consultation, sixteen different cases of bereavement were presented with all participants
presenting at least three times. The fact that over half of the
cases were presented as families may reflect some influence of
the family-systems bias of the consultant, although the clergy
seemed to share at the outset a family orientation. Among the

situations presented were the following: the aftermath of a
non-churched suicide; the delayed grief of an eight year old
boy with both family and school implications; the isolation of
an elderly widow resolved, in part, through the development by
the clergy an of a widow-to-widow support group; difficulties
in working with an alcoholic response to bereavement; psychosomatic ills in response to loss; disintegration and conflict
among mature family members following death of the father; anti-
cipatory grief of the spouse and dying cancer patient; and the
grief of a clergy-participant whose father died during the consultation.

Consistent with the assumption that the clergy are the
most appropriate and natural caretakers of the bereaved, not one
of the participants was rejected by those in whose bereavement
they intervened, even when the clergy were complete strangers
to the bereaved. Only one of the sixteen cases was considered
a "failure" by the members of the consultation. This was the
mature family which disintegrated into three "armed camps" representing three mature children fighting over the elderly widow
who seemed bewildered and helpless as three different clergymen
intervened on behalf of each of the three children and withdrew
assuming that another was the one chosen to resolve the family
feud.

Follow-up questionnaires asking for a general evaluation of
the consultation indicated unanimity of felt-gains in (a) understanding the crisis of bereavement, (b) acquiring new skills for
intervening among the bereaved, and (c) understanding through
group process of one's own attitudes and feelings about death,
dying, and bereavement. All except one of the participants had
experienced the loss through death of at least one close family
member. Each of the participants felt that the direct experience of personal bereavement and the training and experience
as religious functionaries at the time of mourning and grief of
others were the two most influential factors in determing their
attitudes toward the bereaved both prior to and after the consultation.

The consultation was apparently successful in building a
bridge to greater communication and cooperation between the
clergy and the Community Mental Health Center. The extension
of the consultation, for example, was at the request of the
clergy who also expressed a need for consultation on general
mental health problems. Two members of the consultation volun-
teered to serve on the Board of Advisors of the Mental Health
Center. One clergy-intern assisted the Southwest mental health
team in a preventive program for adolescents which eventually
made liberal use of church facilities. In addition to an

increase of referrals to the mental health team from the clergy, there was also an increase of requests by the mental health team for pastoral care and follow-up of the team's clientele.

A multiple-choice type of survey was administered both prior to and following the consultation to assess clergy attitudes and opinions about bereavement and any changes which may, in part, have been attributed to the consultation experience. The results were analyzed by inspection and compared with the published results of two other samples: 125 widows and widowers recently bereaved and a mixed group of 133 professional consultants including physicians, clergy, marriage counselors, psychologists, and nurses (Kutscher, 1969). Prior to the consultation the clergy responses appear to have been more similar to those of the bereaved than to those of the professional consultants. Although the reverse was evident in the post-consultation results, in general, there was good agreement between the responses of the clergy-consultees and those of both the bereaved and professionals. Concurrence with responses of the bereaved sample may support the assumption that the clergy are the closest and most appropriate caretakers of the bereaved, providing an empathic source of comfort, satisfaction, and encouragement. Responses similar to those of the professionals suggest an acceptance among the consultees of the wisdom and knowledge of a group of persons who have taken a special interest in bereavement.

IMPLICATIONS FOR RESEARCH

As with much of the literature on bereavement, this paper is limited in the necessary hard data from which one can generalize. However, the consultation experience did have the heuristic value of discovering and suggesting areas for future research. Within the framework of crisis psychology, the following are some of the hypotheses which could form the basis of a program of research into bereavement: (a) the widowed, in comparison with the married, experience a significantly higher incidence of mental, physical, and psychosomatic illness; (b) preventive and rehabilitative intervention among the bereaved significantly reduces the incidence of negative outcomes as compared with a control group of those in whose bereavement there is no systematic intervention; (c) "normal" grief *does* follow a stereotyped pattern of responses and occurs in stages similar to those outlined in this paper; (d) those who receive intervention counseling during the first few seeks after a significant loss show less morbidity or maladjustment than those who receive assistance at a later time; (e) individuals with

high religious values cope with bereavement more constructively
than do persons with low religious values; (f) followers of
religious traditions with well structured bereavement rituals
including support through the first year of bereavement (*e.g.*,
the Jewish rites and rituals) show less physical and psychological pathology than adherents of religious traditions with
little or no ritual beyond the funeral service (*e.g.*, free
church congregationalists); (g) when one spouse is dying of a
terminal illness, the grief reactions of both the dying and
surviving spouse will yield more constructive outcomes the
higher the degree of openness and interpersonal sharing between the spouses.

Given the avowed goals and concerns of social and behavioral sciences and the inevitability of death to which we
humans must in some way react, it is rather puzzling that, with
a few exceptions, psychologists and sociologists have contributed so little to the bereavement literature. Certainly, the
present dearth of information on bereavement does not reflect
its practical or theoretical importance. Experience of the
consultation reported in this paper suggests that one source
of research information for the community psychologist lies in
greater use of community caretakers. As for bereavement research, caretakers such as the clergy and public health nurses
are rich sources for case-finding and data collecting, and, in
some cases, should be invited to collaborate with us for a more
systematic and thorough research into bereavement.

REFERENCES

Anderson, C.   Aspects of pathological grief and mourning.
International Journal of Psychoanalysis, 1949, *30*, 48-55.

Averill, J. R.   Grief: Its nature and significance.   *Psychological Bulletin*, 1968, 70, *6*, 721-748.

Baler, L. A. & Golde, P. J.   Conjugal bereavement: a strategic
area of research in preventive psychiatry.   Mimeographed
paper.   Bereavement study.   Harvard Medical School, 1964,
1-36.

Barnacle, C.   Grief reactions and their treatment.   *Diseases
of the Nervous System*, 1949, *10*, 173-176.

Bowlby, J.   Grief and mourning in infancy and early childhood.
Psychoanalytic Study of the Child, 1960, *15*, 9-52.

Bowlby, J.   Processes of mourning.   *International Journal of
Psychoanalysis*, 1961, *42*, 317-340.

Bowlby, J.   Pathological mourning and childhood mourning.
Journal of American Psychoanalytic Association, 1963, *11*,
500-541.

Caplan, G.   *Principles of preventive psychiatry*.   New York:
Basic Books, 1964.

Clayton, P., Desmarais, L., & Winokur, G.   A study of normal
bereavement.   A paper presented at the American Psychiatric
Association Meetings, Detroit, Michigan, May 8-12, 1967.

Davis, D. R.   The psychological mechanisms of depressions.   In
E. B. Davies (Ed.), *Depression*.   Cambridge: Cambridge University Press, 1964.

Deutsch, H.   Absence of grief.   *Psychoanalytic Quarterly*, 1937,
6, 12-22.

Feifel, H. (Ed.)   *The meaning of death*.   New York: McGraw-Hill,
1959.

Fleming, J., & Altschul, S.   Activation of mourning and growth
by psychoanalysis.   *International Journal of Psychoanalysis*, 1963, *44*, 419-431.

Freidson, E. Specialties without roots: the utilization of a new service. *Human Organizations,* 1959, *18,* 112-116.

Freidson, E. *Patients' views of medical practice.* New York: Russell Sage Foundation, 1961.

Freud, S. Mourning and melancholia. (Originally published, 1917). In J. Strachey (Ed.), *The standard edition of the complete psychological works of Sigmund Freud,* 14. London: Hogarth, 1957.

Fulton, R. *Death and identity.* New York: John Wiley and Sons, 1965.

Gerber, I. Bereavement and the acceptance of professional services. *Community Mental Health Journal,* 1969, 5, *6,* 487-495.

Gorer, G. *Death, grief, and mourning.* Garden City, New York: Doubleday, 1965.

Greene, W. A. & Miller, G. Psychological factors and reticulo-endothelial disease. *Psychosomatic Medicine,* 1958, *20,* 124-144.

Gurin, G., Veroff, J., & Feld, S. *Americans view their mental health.* New York: Basic Books, 1960.

Hinton, J. *Dying.* Baltimore, Maryland: Penguin Books, 1967.

Irion, P. E. *The funeral and the mourner.* New York: Abingdon, 1954.

Jackson, E. N. *Understanding grief.* New York: Abingdon, 1957.

Jackson, E. N. Grief and religion. In H. Feifel (Ed.), *The meaning of death.* New York: McGraw-Hill, 1959, 218-283.

Jackson, E. N. *For the living.* Des Moines, Iowa: Channel Press, 1963.

Jenson, G. D., & Wallace, J. G. Family mourning process. *Family Press,* 1967, *6,* 56-66.

Kidorf, I. W. Jewish tradition and the Freudian theory of mourning. *Journal of Religion and Health,* 1963, *2,* 248-252.

Kidorf, I. W. The Shiva: a form of group psychotherapy. *Journal of Religion and Health,* 1966, 5, *1,* 43-46.

Kollar, E. Psychological stress. *Journal of Nervous and Mental Disorders*, 1961, *32*, 382-396.

Kraus, A. S., & Lilienfeld, A. M. Some edidemiological aspects of the high mortality rate in the young widowed group. *Journal of Chronic Diseases*, 1959, *10*, 207-217.

Kutscher, A. H. (Ed.) *But not to lose*. New York: Frederick Fell, 1969, Appendix.

Lehrman, R. Reactions to untimely death. *Psychiatric Quarterly* 1956, *30*, 564-578.

Lidz, R. Emotional factors in hyperthyroidism. *Psychosomatic Medicine*, 1949, *11*, 2.

Lieberman, E. J. Americans no longer know how to mourn. *The Washington Post, Potomac*, December 20, 1970, 7-25.

Lindemann, E. Symptomatology and management of acute grief. *American Journal of Psychiatry*, 1944, *101*, 141-148.

Lindemann, E. Modifications in the course of ulcerative colitis in relationship to change in life situations and reaction patterns. *Archives of Research on Nervous and Mental Disease*, 1950, *29*, 706.

MacCurdy, J. T. *The psychology of emotion: Morbid and normal*. London: Kagan Paul, 1925.

Mandelbaum, D. G. Social uses of funeral rites. In H. Feifel (Ed.). *The meaning of death*. New York: McGraw-Hill, 1959, 189-217.

Marris, P. *Widows and their families*. London: Routledge and Kegan Paul, 1958.

McDermott, N., & Cobb, S. Psychogenic factors in asthma. *Psychosomatic Medicine*, 1939, *1*, 204-234.

Mitford, J. *The American way of death*. New York: Simon and Schuster, 1963.

Moreno, J. L. The socialization and death. *Sociometry*, 1947, *10*, 80-84.

Parad, H. J. (Ed.). *Crisis Intervention*. New York: Family Service Association of America, 1965.

Parkes, C. M.   Effects of bereavement on physical and mental health--a study of the medical records of widows. *British Medical Journal*, 1964. *2*, 274-279.

Parkes, C. M.   Grief as an illness. *New Society*, 1964. *3*, 11.

Parkes, C. M.   Bereavement and mental illness. *British Journal of Medical Psychology*, 1965, *38*, 1-26.

Parkes, C. M.   Grief and mourning. *International Journal of Psychoanalysis*, 1967, *3*, 435-438.

Paul, N. L., & Grosser, G. H.   Operational mourning and its role in conjoint family therapy. *Community Mental Health Journal*, 1965, *1*, 339-345.

Peck, M.   Notes on identification in a case of depression reactive to the death of a love object. *Psychoanalytic Quarterly*, 1939, *8*, 1-17.

Rees, W. D., & Lutkins, S. G.   Mortality of bereavement. *British Medical Journal*, 1967, *4*, 13-16.

Rochlin, G.   *Griefs and discontents: The forces of change.* Boston: Little, Brown & Co., 1965.

Roth, M.   The obsessive compulsive condition, the phobic anxiety depersonalization syndrome. *Proceedings of the Royal Society of Medicine*, 1959, *52*, 587-595.

Shoor, M., & Speed, M. H.   Delinquency as a manifestation of the mourning process. *Psychiatric Quarterly*, 1963, *37*, 540-558.

Siggin, L. D.   Mourning: a critical survey of the literature. *International Journal of Psycho-Analysis*, 1966, *47*, 14-25.

Silverman, P. R.   Services to the widowed: first steps in a program of preventive intervention. *Community Mental Health Journal*, 1967, *3*, 37-44.

Stern, K., Williams, G., & Prados, M.   Grief reactions in later life. *American Journal of Psychiatry*, 1951, *108*, 289-294.

Sudnow, D.   *Passing on.*   New Jersey: Prentice-Hall, 1967.

Volkan, V.   Normal and pathological grief reactions. *Virginia Medical Monthly*, 1966, *93*, 651-656.

Volkart, E. H. (Ed.) *Social behavior and personality contributions of W. I. Thomas to theory and social research.* New York: Social Science Research Council, 1951, 12-14.

Woodward, K. L.   How America lives with death. *Newsweek,* April 6, 1970, 75, *14,* 81-88.

Young, M., Benjamin, B., & Wallis, C.   The mortality of widowers. *Lancet,* 1963, 454-456.

11: THE OPPORTUNITY OF THE DRUG CRISIS

In this chapter, Dennis Jaffe presents a striking approach to working with crises engendered by the use of psychedelic drugs. Mr. Jaffe begins by describing the historical and philosophical factors which shape the treatment of drug crises in America. He notes that the public tendency has been to view the "bad trip" experience as an unmitigated disaster and a consequence of moral turpitude. Mr. Jaffe asserts that the consequent intervention strategies have had the effect of denying the drug user the opportunity to benefit by his experience, or of actually increasing his distress. The author then presents a treatment model founded on the idea that the "bad trip" is a true crisis, *i.e.*, may be successfully resolved to the benefit of the individual, and is not merely a catastrophe calling for efforts to minimize damage.

The helping approach described in the paper centers upon the possibility of aiding the tripper to learn and grow from his conflicted feelings. The person in crisis is encouraged to explore and integrate the experiences he has under the drug. Although the method seems to require some sophistication on the part of the help-giver, Mr. Jaffe does not relegate the job to professional mental health workers. Indeed, he argues that professionals often suffer from the cultural bias that lead to destructive methods of intervention. The paper also contains a case history illustrative of the approach being advocated.

THE REPRESSION AND SUPPORT OF PSYCHEDELIC EXPERIENCE

Dennis T. Jaffe

THE STATE STREET CENTER: NUMBER 9

Basic Issues. A 1972 Gallup Poll reports that 20% of the nation's college students have tried psychedelic drugs, up 1800% in the past 4 years, at a time when the government has halted most research on the uses of these drugs as too dangerous, and spends millions of dollars to control their use. In the controversy that has lasted a decade the powerful interests which have led to these policies effectively counter the demands of well over a million young people to use these drugs. The controversy concerns the usefulness and validity of the experiences people report with these drugs, and whether American society will allow change in the area of personal experience. Psychedelic drugs are powerful and unpredictable, and sometimes result in difficulties which need medical or crisis intervention. Help must be offered within the value context of the drug user, or else the helper runs the risk of reflecting the prejudices and fears of current drug policies, which are plainly against the interests of those who use the drugs. The nature of this conflict of interests is the theme of this paper.

Willis Harman, an engineering professor turned psychedelic researcher (and now turned future-caster), clearly defined the gap between policy and reality as long ago as 1963:

> The consciousness-expanding drugs LSD and psilocybin have been hailed, in some quarters at least, as having fantastic potentialities for aiding man to know himself, for helping him release his creative powers, for contributing toward reducing his alienation from himself and his fellow man and toward the discovery and creation of meaning in his life. Yet LSD was recently banned in Canada, along with thalidomide, as a "dangerous drug," and in general it is harder to get than heroin or cyanide. ...Dr. Sidney Cohen, who has made what are no doubt the most detailed studies of adverse reactions to LSD, recently summarized his findings in

159

the statement, "Considering the enormous scope of
the psychic responses it induces, LSD is an aston-
ishingly safe drug." Physiologically, it is less
dangerous than aspirin or penicillin, and certainly
far less deleterious than alcohol or tobacco. Yet
a recent editorial in the psychiatric organ of the
AMA warns that "greater sickness and even death is
in store...unless controls are developed against the
unwise use of LSD," and expresses alarm that the
public has heard of the claimed benefits from LSD
and "is looking for psychiatrists who specialize in
its administration." (Harman, 1963, P. 5)

In 1966 Harman's center at Stanford University, in the midst of
detailed studies of therapy and creativity with LSD which initially showed highly promising results, along with all but two
other research centers had its license to use LSD terminated.

Evidently the threat of LSD arouses some powerful defensive
reactions in society. While professional judgment is invoked to
justify each step of social policy, the issues raised by psychedelics involve matters of values and ethics. Against this background, therapists have to intervene with individual users in
difficulty. Even these interventions are colored by where the
helper stands on these issues. For example, if one considered
the experience of psychedelics potentially useful one would help
out differently than if one considered the effects harmful and
aimed only at stopping them. Crisis intervention thus depends
on an understanding of the nature of psychedelics, and the controversy surrounding them.

Peak Experience and Value Change. The sudden shift of young
people from alcohol to marijuana (a mild psychedelic), LSD, mes-
caline, peyote, psilocybin and other psychedelics can only be explained when their unique nature is explicated. Since young
people value these drugs enough to risk criminal penalties and
poisonous impurities, they must do something different or better
than alcohol. Drug policies try to account for the shift with
simplistic theories of peer group pressure and rebellion, and exclude the possibility that psychedelic use may in some ways represent positive and useful activity.

Psychedelic drug use is only one aspect of a shift in values
and priorities which has occurred among young people. Slater
and others suggest that this incipient counter culture differs in
the following ways from the prevailing culture:

The old culture, when forced to choose, tends to give
preference to property rights over personal rights,
technological requirements over human needs, competition

over cooperation, violence over sexuality, concentration over distribution, the producer over the consumer,
means over ends, secrecy over personal openness, social
forms over personal expression, striving over gratifi-
cation, Oedipal love over communal love, and so on.
The counter culture tends to reverse all these priorities. (Slater, 1970; p. 100)

Drug use is a form of the search to change oneself, and
form new kinds of relationships to oneself, others, and society.
The growing use of psychedelics would be explained if the experiences with these drugs, *help young people to reach their goals.*
The best way to explain the shift from alcohol to psychedelics
by a large number of intelligent and aware young people is that
it helped them get where they wanted to go. Psychedelics seem
to catalyze experiences which are at times, quite valuable and
useful, and which are not peculiar to the drug, but are characteristic of a more general class of growth experiences.

There are experiences which are so profound and impressive
that they result in new orientations towards basic values, relations toward others and oneself. Such remarkable and historically rare events are called religious, mystical, transcendental
or mad, and are not typically seen as having great practical or
social significance, other than to the extent that they led to
religious communities, as with the conversion of St. Paul.
Abraham Maslow, one of the few psychologists to look at healthy
rather than pathological human functioning, reports that such
events have much in common with the aesthetic, oceanic, creative,
loving, therapeutic, parental, orgasmic, athletic or intellectual experiences where his respondents report they are most themselves, most in touch with who they are, and most alive and productive in terms of their basic values. Healthy people report
these peak experiences more commonly and frequently than average
people. Such experiences are:

an episode, or a spurt in which the powers of the person come together in a particularly efficient and intensely enjoyable way, and in which he is more integrated and less split, more open for experience, more
idiosyncratic, more perfectly expressive or spontaneous, or fully functioning, more creative, more humor-
ous, more ego-transcending, more independent of his
lower needs, etc. He becomes in these episodes more
truly himself, more perfectly actualizing his poten-
tialities, closer to the core of his Being. (Maslow,
1962; p. 91)

The cumulative evidence of research is that psychedelics,
when used under carefully supervised conditions, enormously

increases the probability and frequency of such peak experiences.
Wilson Van Dusen, who has given LSD to chronic alcoholics, says:

> There is a central human experience which alters all
> other experiences...it is the very heart of human
> experience. It is the center that gives understand-
> ing to the whole. It has been called Satori in
> Japanese Zen, moksha in Hinduism, religious enlight-
> enment or cosmic consciousness in the West....LSD
> appears to facilitate the discovery of this central
> human experience. (Van Dusen, 1961; p. 11)

Stanislav Grof, a psychoanalyst in Prague, used small doses
of LSD in repeated sessions (up to 80 in all, at weekly intervals) with his most disturbed neurotic and psychotic patients.
In data gathered over a decade of work, he details how psychedelics enormously increase the range and depth of therapy, while
decreasing the time needed for it, in cases which had not previously responded to any kind of treatment. According to Grof,
psychedelics magnify anything that happens to a person: his perceptions, fears, expectations and inner feelings. By placing
one in touch with repressed and primitive material of consciousness, psychedelics can be quite frightening.

Initially, many therapists were confused and unsettled by
the strange and novel reactions to this new class of drugs.
Unger reports that this was particularly true of those who did
not themselves take LSD. He points out that peak experiences
could easily be described, and devalued, by psychoanalysts as
"delusionary escapes from unresolved infantile or Oedipal conflicts." The description of LSD as primarily anxiety or psychosis producing was based on observation not balanced by personal
experience. Savage and Stolaroff suggest some reasons why professionals would resist the usefulness of psychedelics:

> The hallucinogens (more properly called psychedlic
> agents when used to explore new understanding of the
> mind) open up dimensions of consciousness with which
> few therapists are familiar. The heightened sensi-
> tivity and enhancement of sensory modalities, the re-
> living of events in time and other dimensionless
> phenomena, and the oft-reported profound philosophic
> and universal experiences, tend to lie outside the
> therapists' conceptual frame of reference. ...Con-
> trary to the belief of many investigators, the hal-
> lucinogens do not produce experiences but inhibit
> repressive mechanisms that ordinarily allow sub-
> jects to explore the contents of their own minds.
> (Savage and Stolaroff, 1965; p. 218)

The extent and direction of the changes in patients reported by Grof go far beyond the outcome of traditional therapeutic procedures, and thus are another source of the uneasiness which has accompanied reports of psychedelic research. A few of the outcomes he mentiones are:

> The patients who have reported deep experiences of melted ecstacy in these advanced sessions showed very specific changes in perception of themselves and the world, in their behavior and their hierarchy of values. As a rule, psychopathological symptoms were greatly reduced--depression dissolved, anxiety and tension disappeared, guilt feelings were lifted. Deep feelings of relaxation, serenity, tranquility and inner peace seemed to be the rule....The self image was greatly improved and an enhanced feeling of health and smooth physiological functioning was very common....They became more understanding, empathic and living toward their fellowman and perceived the world as a fascinating and basically friendly place....The subjects were discovering meaning and beauty in ordinary things of their everyday environment....There was a more definite need for personal freedom and the antiauthoritarian tendencies were definitely increased. The previously all important values seemed trivial (striving for power, status, money, fame, etc.) and a deep wisdom was discovered in simplicity of life....These true values (sense for beauty, love, justice, etc.) were accepted readily and joyfully as part of the universal order rather than because of fear of punishment. There seems to be a striking parallel here with Maslow's findings in people who had spontaneous peak experiences. Many of the mentioned attitudes can be found in an extreme form in the hippie movement, sometimes exaggerated to the point of caricature. (Grof, 1972; Pp 218-219)

Grof's work suggests some fascinating connections. LSD therapy has produced results in mental patients in Prague, which correspond almost precisely to Maslow's Being values (which he feels are basic, natural, human and good as reported by healthy, fully functioning people), and to the values of hippies and other young people. Grof's results could not have been produced as a result of his expectations, because he only learned of Maslow, Jung and other depth psychologists when his traditional psychoanalytic formulations could no longer account for what he was seeing. He is now director of one of the two extant psychedelic therapy centers in the U.S., and ironically works under greater restrictions than he faced in Prague.

There have been over 1,000 studies of psychedelics, and most of them suggest positive effects following its use. The evidence of research teams all over the world is that not only does LSD help alleviate traditional symptoms, but it also tends to lead to a change in values and goals. It can effect a total personality reorganization, even in a single administration. Studies of single massive doses, with alcoholics, terminal cancer patients and neurotic patients all have shown positive results, where other interventions are ineffective, or in the case of terminal cancer patients, nonexistent. There is clearly a tremendous disparity between research results, and government accounts of the lack of available data, and the danger of supervised psychedelic use.

Illegal Users and the New Culture. If there is any veracity in previous research, then it can be predicted that psychedelic use by young people should have powerful positive and negative effects. Since such experimentation is done without the safeguards and controls of research settings, it can also be expected that dangers which are avoided in clinical settings will crop up in nonsanctioned use. But to the extent that use is informed by the conditions for safe and proper experiences, the results can also be highly positive. The frequency of positive reports by young people, and the similarity of psychedelic therapy changes and certain aspects of the youth culture, suggests that positive results of psychedelic use are causes as well as results of the development of a new culture by youth.

I am presently part of a research team collecting life histories from young psychedelic users in five parts of the country. Two hour interviews focus on their experiences with drugs, how they came to use them, and the ways that drug use affected their relations to themselves, family, friends, lovers, school, society and basic values. The accounts shed much doubt on the hysterical and negative stories which dot medical and media outlets. With full knowledge of the risks, young people choose to use psychedelics for the same reasons that researchers study them. They rarely seem disappointed. Also, they rarely use psychedelics more often than weekly during an initial stage of not more than a few months. Temperance and moderation are the rule, because they are regarded as learning tools, not as escapist fare or pleasure drugs, and are treated with great respect. Ironically, youthful psychedelic users exhibit the good judgment, awareness of both sides of the issue, utilization of real data and others' experiences, reflection on the experience and desire for corroboration and exchange that are the earmarks of the scientific method, and completely lacking in some of the more professional accounts and opinions on drug use.

Our 150 respondents represent a crossection of youth by age,

present drug use (still users or discontinued) and positive and
negative effects (many have been hospitalized or arrested on
account of drug use, and almost all report on bad trips). They
overwhelmingly assess their experiences as positive, and detail
the specific stages of learning and growth as corresponding to
different types of drug use. They see the changes as in the
direction of their goals, and see their values as different from
the dominant culture and as shared with other young people around
them. They report great pain and struggle in their attempts to
change, and report that misuse or overuse of psychedelics can be
disastrous. They respond positively to marijuana, hashish, which
they use frequently, and the stronger psychedelics which are used
less often, and associate them with personality and value changes.
Alcohol, amphetamines, barbiturates and tranquillizers are used,
but for more traditional results such as tension release, avoidance of negative feelings, and relaxation, and are mentioned as
quite different from psychedelics.

Psychedelics are most usefully used as part of a conscious
growth process, which extends both before and after the trip.
One girl tells of her most significant psychedelic experience.

> One that was by myself. I don't think consciously of
> working on something when I trip, but that one time I
> did, and that was right after I had moved out from
> living with A. I went to the beach. I remember feel-
> ing alone at first, but then it was really good. I
> like to be out in nature. That one time was the only
> time I ever did it specifically to work on something.
> I find that things usually work out in my head anyway,
> but I don't do it deliberately. I do it in the process
> of watching an ant. I trip to play and for kind of
> spiritual enlightenment, and as a vacation kind of
> thing. With drugs, it is a kind of religious exper-
> ience out in the woods to have a feeling of oneness,
> to feel a part of life and life processes. It doesn't
> seem supernatural. It's just natural and awesome.
> Being humbled. I don't think that consciously about
> it, but it has something to do with putting things in
> perspective. It's standing back from all that and re-
> alizing that our world's not going to fall apart if you
> don't get to the grocery store today. You can have
> that experience just by getting away and taking a vaca-
> tion, but drugs seem to heighten that for me.

Another girl reports not much learning or change from scores of
experiences with many drugs, until:

> I never conceptualized any of my drug use until last
> year. The first one which we really planned was with B.

> We got real close and played music, and then we went
> to a plastic shopping center and realized that it was
> just that, a plastic bourgeois shopping center. I
> reached a whole new level. I was coming from think-
> ing of things in a linear and culturally determined
> fashion to a much more intuitive way. I realized
> that I didn't have to think all the time and read.
> I could rely on my intuition. I had gotten into a
> pattern or trap, and the acid destroyed me so I could
> build up things again.

That too is a stage, and the level she is at is unstable and she
later returns to the school she had left:

> I had started an intentional process to de-intellectual-
> ize myself, but I got caught in all kinds of clichés
> and couldn't express myself articulately, so I'm back
> in school and getting my mind to work again.

Young people have a tremendous psychological sophistication,
stemming largely from reading combined with their familiarity
with inner experience. When a bad experience occurs, the person
often knows himself well enough to work on correcting it so that
the next experience will be better. The concepts of therapeutic
working through are in everyday usage among young people:

> I first had mescaline in a country gathering. It
> wasn't a great trip. My girlfriend and I dropped
> and all this stuff we'd been repressing came out.
> My visual image of it was this violent stranglchold
> on each other, and we couldn't let go, we were frozen
> there. Getting stoned made the whole thing come out
> in high relief. It's now my conviction that either
> it's a mistake to do psychedelics wanting something,
> or one has to be very careful about how one sets
> one's mind to want something. Or else what the trip
> is about is the thing that you want tortures you.

> After I started doing psychedelics I was really re-
> lentless about trying to make it work. My first
> good trip happened when I dropped mescaline in the
> airport. It was like every trip before had been a
> resistance which wasn't going with the flow. And
> then I had this amazing experience while I was eat-
> ing breakfast of hearing this beautiful music. At
> first I thought it was coming out of the headset,
> but it was coming out of my head. It was taking the
> sounds of the engine and transforming them into a
> musical score. And then I found that I could trans-
> form the music, highlighting the brass section, etc.

And it really made me ecstatic, a bonafide ecstatic
experience! And then I looked out the window and
noticed the earth was breathing.

That had a profound effect on me. I've since been
empowered by the practice of "facing things." I
guess I learned that I had this emotional body I had
to liberate, and the only way to liberate it was by
facing reality. Drugs played a big part by putting
me in touch with ecstacy. And it was also manifest
to me that ecstacy and pain exist along the same
vector of sensation. And if you've got pain stored
up in your body, then the only way to experience
ecstasy is to experience it through the pain.

Another subject reports working through a conflict by fantasy:

It was about that time that I got eaten by this big
red mouth. I was making love on acid and got eaten.
At first it was horrible, but then I got eaten and
that was that. It felt like some kind of symbolic
turning point. But drugs were taking the lid off of
a sexual repression, among a whole group of people that
I was with all the time.

He speaks of drugs as accentuating the sense of communal sharing,
and others report instances of telepathic union of a couple or
group. On the negative side, the increased sensitivity to others
and the environment also produces heightened perception of fears.
Since drug use is illegal, many report paranoia and fears of
getting caught are accentuated. To escape this, and to move
toward the union with the earth and nature which many psychedelic
users desire, many people eventually move to the country for a
period of their lives:

We were all outlaws and the paranoia levels were rampant. But most of the time you knew who your friends
were because of the solidarity of drugs. In the moun-
tains there was less paranoia and drugs were different.
You could consume less and still stay on top of ordinary reality. I went from feeling I had no roots to
seeing them everywhere and feeling caught in them.
Things were no longer flat any more. It gave a dimension to my existence and liberated energy.

He expressed his discovery of the social basis of mankind through
work in a form of mythic theatre troupe.

Another account is from a middle-aged architect who went
through a period of great change with psychedelics:

> I've never taken them as uppers or downers. I've
> taken them to play, but it always is an experiment
> cuz I never know what's going to happen. Mostly I
> take them as an edge, to break patterns. I don't
> ever take them when I don't feel good. A couple
> of years ago I was going through a lot of ambival-
> ence about commitment to women, and I lived up here
> alone for a month. I'd smoke a lot of dope and it
> bummed me all the time. Bummers, were being afraid
> of just about everything; machines, hating everything
> I'd designed, hating myself for ever having cut down
> a tree, being afraid about people. I think that dope
> blasted me out of roles and perceptions that were
> keeping me tied in. It was catalytic, it changed
> motivation, my whole future orientation. All those
> things I used to worry about.

Sometimes people report changes which might be regarded as
negative, even though they feel them as positive:

> Another thing that has happened is that I am very
> inarticulate most of the time. I am just not able
> to think and talk in a linear way any more. I am
> not able to make complex plans any more. That's
> right on for me.

Prolonged or frequent use seems to result in negative changes
which are not reported in the research literature. These include
confusion, disorientation, and a general dullness caused by the
overstimulation of the trips. Material which comes up is defended against, and the subject seems to develop all the defenses
to psychedelic experience which are characteristic of everyday
experience. At this point the person either chooses to stop
using drugs or cut down drastically, or else switches to a more
alienating type of drug, from heroin, to speed to barbiturates.
The intensity and vitatility of psychedelics soon fade.

> I thought, hey, wait a minute man, I'm never going
> to get my shit together if I don't stop this for
> awhile. For one thing my memory was getting really
> fucked up. I couldn't remember anything. My, world
> was just always on a trip, you know. My life was
> just one long trip it seemed. I wasn't living in
> the real world at all. My world was all fantasy.
> I couldn't hold on to anything-everything was just
> slipping through my fingers and I felt that I had
> to stop tripping so much. That whole period of my
> life is a haze now.

Like many others, she found a community that would offer the support that she needed, and began to be more involved with others. She found that she could explore experience and express herself much better in a community than ever on drugs. She now feels she understands the door-opening qualities of psychedelics, and uses them only infrequently when she knows she can handle and has the time to deal with what comes up.

The preceding are an almost random sample of the literally thousands of anecdotes which document the richness, variety and creativity with which young people are using psychedelics. The positive experiences and people who have grown greatly outnumber the few who use drugs self-destructively. Also, much of our data suggests that most self-destructive drug use is an episode, a stage of growth, which leads to so much pain that it eventually transcends itself, usually to a level of greater insight and more productive use of energies. There is a great deal of accumulated learning among young people, about themselves, personal change and change experiences such as drugs and new communities, but its underground nature has kept this data from most professional circles.

To sum up, there are several categories which cover the uses which young people make of psychedelics. They are:

1. *Getting into the here and now.* This is also the goal of sensitivity groups and Gestalt therapy, and is experienced as a corrective to the cognitive, detached, patterned way in which people are taught to deal with the world. This is usually connected with a discovery of the body, and sensual and sense pleasures. Patterns break down, and free flowing consciousness dazzles one with creative new patterns.

2. *To see something real, vivid, novel, exciting.* The major educational experience that young people report is boredom and sensory deprivation. They feel a need to blast themselves into experience, to saturate themselves with something new, to make up for that. This can be an end in itself, or a spur to new kinds of experiencing and activity.

3. *Exploring consciousness and the inner self.* This is the journey associated with psychoanalysis, madness and artistic creation. The change is that archetypal and repressed experience is experienced in fantasy and lived through, and eventually loses its fearsomeness. Jung and Norman O. Brown guide this trip much better than Freud. There is a growing interest in rituals, other cultures, and extraordinary states of consciousness. There is a renewed

or more vivid experience of feelings, and a sensitivity to the ambivalence characteristic of all relationships.

4. *To end anxiety and boundaries between people and
   parts of oneself.* The goal is to achieve unity and
   to end alienation which has been self-induced by
   the culture. Communities and relationships are
   organic wholes, and are natural and not to be feared.
   The fear and anxiety which accompanies this trip is
   a culturally determined defense which can be system-
   matically reduced as one achieves wholeness.

5. *To achieve transcendence, Satori, peak experience.*
   The search for higher states of consciousness usually starts with psychedelics, but eventually leads
   to one of the older traditional religious disciplines,
   like meditation, Tai Chi, yoga or speaking in tongues.
   The goal is to get high and to maintain the state,
   which cannot be done except for moments with drugs.

Society Defends Against Psychedelic Learning. Evidence for
the safety and potential of psychedelics has been presented from
research and the experience of young people. Why has society reacted so negatively to them? Simplistic reactions scapegoat the
messianic claims and proselytizing of figures like Tim Leary,
and the extreme cases of supposed "bad trips" and even deaths,
which are largely unrecorded in medical literature, to justify
repressive policies against all use. Since there is no similar
reaction to the thousands of alcohol-caused body deteriorations,
violent incidents and auto accidents, it is wise to consider
alternate explanations for the powerful negative reaction.

There is evidence that psychedelics greatly increase the
frequency and likelihood of peak experiences, which are not only
"self-validating, self-justifying moments which carry their own
intrinsic value with them" (Maslow), but seem to have long-lasting and therapeutic effects, and facilitate personality and value
change. Young people use psychedelics to explore themselves and
their world. Maslow points out that those having frequent peak
experiences have different priorities around the basic values of
life. This value system is similar to Buddhist and Eastern
philosophy, as well as the youth counter culture. These values
run into conflict with the values of the dominant culture, and
lead to the backlash which young people and psychedelics face.

The dominant culture devalues and avoids exploration of
inner experience, and concentrates on mastery of the external
world and control over the self. The dimensions of the conflict

are old and well traveled, and Slater's dichotomies are only the most recent manifestation. Sided with today's dominant culture is the recent prophet Freud, who felt that civilization was a precarious balance in which creative and ordering forces of the ego overcame the aggressive and self-destructive forces of the id. Political theorists Hobbes and Locke locate the safety of society in contracts which people enter for their protection, and see man in need of rulers and laws to maintain control over his bad inner self.

The opposite view is that man is naturally in harmony with nature and himself, and has nothing to fear from the natural impulses, death, and disorder. It is the cornerstone of Eastern thought, and has been formulated in the West by Maslow, Jung, Hesse, Laing, Rousseau and in Plato's later dialogues. One view is that man should strive for greater control over himself and his inner experience, as is personified by the order, rigidity, secrecy, drabness and unresponsiveness of the Nixon administration. The other view is that inner experience should flow naturally and be expressed as unity with nature, and that man can thus attain higher ranges of Being and consciousness. Each theory has masses of evidence to support its claims, and the adoption of one or the other seems to be a matter of personal and cultural temperament. But psychedelics evidently lead to conversions from the predominant to the alternative viewpoint, and thus are potentially subversive.

There are currently great strains on the system of tight control, which seems on the verge of demonstrating its alienation from nature by destroying it. Advocates of closer control, which cuts man further off from the experience and natural values which could bring him back into touch, lead to a self-defeating spiral. Anxiety increases because man is split ever wider. The anxiety is from the gap between man and his inner experience. Psychedelics threaten the dominant culture because their fear of themselves, based on their distance from theselves, leads to the fantasy that they will release something awful from the soul. Youthful drug users accentuate this by being alert to the potential redemptive powers of their experience. They want to see people get in touch with their basic fears, so that they will see their illusory nature, and be less destructive. Opponents of this cannot see beyond the threat to any potential gains, so that the psychedelic claims come out as messianic nonsense. The vehemence and irrationality of the public response can only be explained on the basis of what people fear about themselves.

The mechanisms whereby a culture avoids feelings by placing them in others are documented by Kai Erikson (*Wayward Puritans*), Thomas Szasz (*The Manufacture of Madness*) and R. D. Laing.

Erikson and Szasz study religious persecution, with Szasz extending the parallel to current treatment of mental illness. They make use of a cultural form of the psychoanalytic mechanism of projection. When someone sees another have a feeling or acting in ways that he denies or avoids in himself, he is embarrassed, uncomfortable or angry. When such reactions are shared throughout a culture, that form of behavior is labelled deviant and prohibited with sanctions. Deviants call into question values upon which the culture has agreed, and must be discouraged in order to maintain a shared defense. Szasz cites the treatment of homosexuals as sick or criminal as a mechanism for dealing with the culture's repressed homosexual feelings, by projecting them on the helpless offenders who are caught, and getting rid of them by confinement or psychaitric treatment.

The experiential account of this projection process begins when someone sees an odd action, say a young person dressed differently and doing things which make him uncomfortable, like hugging his friends in the street. He feels that if he acted that way it would mean that he had lost self-control, because a part of him would really like to do that. He then projects, by assuming that any person acting that way has lost self-control. He jumps to the conclusion, based on his view of man as inherently destructive, that when control is gone violent harm will result. This fear on the part of teachers results in regimented classes, strong discipline and hall passes, all aimed at teaching youngsters good control. Yet when this same fear takes the form of feeling that vague others are out to destroy one, it is labelled paranoia. Fears must have culturally sanctioned objects, like the Russians. Fear leads to social control, whether or not this fear has a real basis in the behavior of the other. Laing's *Knots* documents many aspects of mutual projection and the confusing tangle that can result from acting on them. The argument that if drugs are legalized, people will be stoned all the time and all sorts of horrors will result is based on fantasy fears. There is no reason to suppose that legalizing something which millions are doing already will result in an increase in anything, and certainly nothing worse than the self-destructive aspects of drug users distrust of each other and fear of getting caught. The crucial issue for sensible social policies is the decision about whether deviant behavior causes *actual harm to others*. Punishment for lateness to class and for dropping acid are similar in that they do not protect society from harm, but rather protect it from something it might wish to do.

This mechanism is also common in mental hospitals, where people whose actions do not make sense are sent, on the assumption that they are really asking for help. Help is offered in the form of aids to control--locking the mad person up, giving him electric shocks and drugs to calm him down, and trying to

convince him to act differently through therapy. Only heretical
therapists like Laing, who understand that madness is also within themselves, look within the reality of the mad person to
learn how he makes sense out of the world. Projection of fears
also operates when therapists attempt to stop "bad trips" merely
because the person seems highly emotional, inexplicably involved
or upset. The response is always to stop him, control him with
drugs, because it is immediately assumed that his goal is to
terminate the experience. From the previous discussion, it is
more likely that the person would want to continue the trip,
with the aid of someone whose interest is not control.

The dominant culture prefers drugs which either do nothing
to experience, like tobacco, or those which cut one off from
feelings and tension, like tranquillizers and alcohol. The pressure of living creates the need to avoid the intensity of built
up negative feelings. In work and school relations, the usual
norm is that feelings are not relevant, and are counter productive if not kept to ourselves. The poker face is a value; one
does not show pain, anger, sadness and above all fear. The
risks that are encouraged show still more about the culture's
orientation to inner experience. The dangers of a flight to the
moon, which demand steel-hard, emotionless automatons able to
keep cool and calculate under great pressure, skilled in all manner of control technology, create its heroes. The risk of in-
jury in a football game, which is almost certain in a scholastic
career and usually permanent, is sanctioned and applauded, because it models toughness and coolness under pressure.

The risks sanctioned by creating audiences to watch them
define the skills valued by the dominant culture--control, technology, competition, exploitation, power, strength, and emotion-
lessness. Feelings other than well-channeled anger at the other
team, the enemy, are harmful. This is the model that has been
internalized to deal with all conflicts--working together to
overcome a common enemy. It might be better to devise games
where at least part of the enemy is within. Since really we are
not all good and the enemy is not all bad, win/lost strategies
are self-defeating, as our foreign policy continually shows.

With such an orientation it is easy to see why the possible
gain of self-knowledge through psychedelics, when balanced
against the risks of bad feelings and unpleasantness, is not
valued. Thousands die from alcohol, yet LSD is feared. Alcohol
seems socially useful, because it releases violence while it
tranquillizes other feelings, such as closeness to others, leading to the preferred stance for our culture. When faced with
the difficulty of proving harm to others, policy makers end up
having to justify prohibition of psychedelics on the grounds of
the user's possible harm to himself. Such logic could lead to

prohibition of sex for causing neurosis. By appearing to worry about the poor user, who is put in jail or hospital, society avoids its fear mingled with desire of being seduced by drugs. Worry about chromosomes (decisively disproven), psychosis, falling out windows (a real danger, but one which there are other ways to prevent), are mobilized to support current policies.

The danger of possible psychosis must be clarified further. Originally, the LSD experience was classified as a model psychosis, and therapists were urged to try to experience madness. Later studies show that while there are many similarities, in language construction, involvement in fantasy oriented behavior at a symbolic level, and particularly when the expectation is to become psychotic, on other dimensions the experiences are opposite. For example, psychosis is rarely pleasant, and rarely leads to spontaneous personality alteration or growth. Psychosis rather stems from a longstanding invalidation of oneself as a person, so that the sense of oneself and reaction to ego loss in the two modes are quite different. Psychosis is a defensive strategy against the experience of pain in relation to others, while psychedelic experience is often a destructuring of defenses. Psychotic episodes do occur after use of psychedelics, but in each case documented there were clear pre-psychotic personality features. The psychedelic may have precipitated the episode, but previous stability makes such breakdowns highly amenable to even traditional treatments. Also, it has been suggested that crazy people seem to be attracted to psychedelics, so statistics on freakouts may reflect this preference rather than the action of the drug. Grof and Cohen, among others, claim that psychedelics are useful in helping people back after breakdowns. Psychedelic therapists do not fear such breaks, because they see them as treatable and as possible steps in a natural restructuring of consciousness.

Opposition to psychedelics leads to social policies which confuse moral with medical issues, in order to mystify moralistic judgments with medical justification. Morally, the issue is whether people are free to inject drugs they choose. American norms and laws say yes, for some drugs with some limits. Social and medical experience is then considered to regulate conditions where drug use can lead to harm to others, as with drunken driving. The traditional, conservative, civil libertarian, strict constructionist view, shared by most young people whether or not they use drugs, is that limits should only result from the need to protect others.

The rising power of psychiatry led to a further consideration which is the source of current controversy and repression around psychedelics. The moral issue is whether the law should determine, presumably by relying on objective scientific evidence,

what is good for the individual, and enforce that decision. Increasingly the conflict of interests that such judgment might
entail is ignored. Involuntary hospitalization, criminal penalties and enforced treatment for addicts (independently of whatever crimes they may have committed), and the ban on cigarette
commercials on TV are all areas where society tries to protect
its citizens from themselves, and are all ineffective. More
importantly, the first two can happen against the will of the
individual involved, and involuntary hospitalization can happen
without even due process.

Medical authorities justify prohibition on the grounds of
potential harm to the user. He is defined as being ill and requiring treatment merely because of his use of drugs. Treatment has the goal of pursuading the patient to stop using illegal drugs, usually in exchange for prescribed ones. This policy
is in effect the substitution of one group's preference for
psychedelics or heroin, by socially acceptable drugs of proven
harmfulness, like tranquillizers, methodone, alcohol and tobacco.
Among young people, the result of this policy has usually been
that they use both kinds of drugs simultaneously, with nobody
gaining except the policymakers in money and prestige. Because
they utilize the coercive methods of the dominant culture and
refuse to recognize the existence of a conflict of values, current drug policies not only fail to pursuade young people to
cut down on drug use, but also fail to reach and help the obvious casual ties of drug use among young people. All conflicts
have been resolved in favor of the dominant culture, without so
much as a hearing to entertain the interests of young drug
users.

Crisis Intervention with "Bad Trips." The effects of a
psychedelic, say Savage and Stolaroff (1965).

> will depend on a) the mental content, the subject's
> individual personality, conditioning, attitudes,
> values and beliefs; b) his preparation for the ex-
> perience, which determines in part how he will use
> the opportunity; and c) his environment during the
> experience, which very appreciably affects how he
> will deal with the material he touches on and the
> opportunities afforded. Most investigators now
> agree that preparation and setting profoundly affect
> the subject's experience, and the presence of sup-
> portive, understanding, accepting companions is es-
> sential to a comfortable and rewarding session (Pp. 218-221).

Distrust of the experience, lack of a guide, or anxiety induc-
tion from companions or a setting which triggers negative feelings

are some of the aspects of the set and setting of the drug trip which can produce the intense anxiety which is called "bad." Essentially, an intervention must aim at helping the person back to a space where the fear is manageable, and the person can deal with and integrate the experience afterwards without constructing stronger defenses against what the trip has revealed.

The behavior of a tripper is often highly emotional, with shifts of mood and sudden bursts of energy which can be strange and fearsome to someone not used to such activity. Humphrey Osmond, the researcher who coined the term "psychedelic", propounded the controversial Golden Rule, than anyone dealing with psychedelics should start with himself. Unger points out that researchers who overestimated the harmfulness of the psychic reaction to psychedelics were invariably those who did not try the drug themselves. He suggests that the anxiety shown by their subjects may have been induced by their similar feelings. Projection of something is operating when therapists label trips "bad" even though they may lead to rewarding, growth producing personal experiences. The inexperience and negative setting of most hospitals clearly contributes to the bad experiences which young people report when taken there on trips. Savage and Stolaroff suggest:

> By denying these new dimensions of consciousness, or attempting to restrict the experience to his own theoretical framework, the therapist can produce great conflict in the subject, and cause him to reject important parts of the experience or force him into delusional solutions. (Savage & Stolaroff, 1965, Pp. 218-221).

Trips are commonly judged bad on the basis that the tripper was huddled in a corner, crying, screaming or talking to someone who wasn't there. Bad is the discharge of feelings out of context, which threatens some therapists.

Psychedelic therapists agree that harmful effects of a trip are negligable if the drug is used in a comfortable setting, with a guide the user knows and trusts, who has experience both with the drug and as a helper. Sidney Cohen, former drug abuse director of the National Institute of Mental Health, finds almost no record of permanent harm in a 1960 study of 25,000 supervised trips. Grof claims that none of the thousands of trips he has guided, many with the sickest possible people, has led to harm. When a patient had a particularly frightening experience, Grof always found that it was due to unconscious material struggling for recognition. His procedure was to as the patient to trip again as soon as possible to face the fear rather than avoid it. Blewett, in *the Frontiers of Being*, writes that he gave patients more psychedelic when they ran into scary material, and that facilitated the material working into consciousness.

Medical practice tends to devalue the possibilities and reduce the question of bad trips to alleviation of symptoms. This
trend is shown in one of the few articles on the subject, written by Drs. Taylor, Maurer and Tinklenberg in the July 20, 1970
issue of the *Journal of the American Medical Association*. A
month previously in the same journal, Pahnke, Kurland, Unger,
Savage and Grof (the only legal psychedelic therapy team in the
U.S.) wrote about their work. They detailed the special characteristics of LSD, the wide range of experiences possible--psy-
chotic, cognitive, aesthetic, psychodynamic and mystical, and
its possibilities for growth and personality change. Evidently
without benefit of this article, "Management of 'Bad Trips' in
an Evolving Drug Scene" defines the psychedelic experience only
as "producing perceptual and cognitive distortions which, in the
majority of instances are experienced by an individual as strange
but tolerable, if not pleasant or even exhilarating."

The article betrays all the prejudices of the dominant culture. The therapeutic goal is managing the bad trip, which is
"a state of panic varying from mild apprehension to panic," the
exact cause of which is unknown (to the authors at least). They
seek to stop this negative experience, to protect the tripper
from himself and others, the standard medical caveat. They suggest two methods--the preferred one of talking the tripper down,
or sedation. By condoning this second method, the authors be-
tray their total lack of psychological considerations. Thera-
peutically, sedation of a tripper amounts to no intervention at
all. Interrupting someone in mid-trip interrupts the natural
process of working on the material which enters consciousness.
It leaves the subject confused, detached, and unable to get back
in touch with what was happening. Since he has lost access to
unconscious material, but is left with the mood it placed him
in, perhaps anxiety or incredulousness, sedation promises an outcome of great difficulty in working through and understanding
the significance of the trip, which is crucial to the outcome.
Sedation is also not warranted, because young people themselves
have discovered that large doses of niacin bring one down quite
gently, without loss of consciousness and subsequent difficulty
in reintegrating and reorienting. Since consciousness is the
working part of the person tripping, no intervention should de-
prive him of its use.

One of the research interviews, with an 18 year old girl,
offers a description of the kind of aid which is more desirable:

> Acid can be used in a really good way, I really truly
> believe. What acid does I think is open a lot of
> doors in your head and lets a lot of things out. I just

had so many repressed feelings that when I did acid
it opened these doors and things came out that I just
wasn't really ready to handle. I was going through
heavy things with my parents. They were freaked out
about the things I was doing, really put across the
idea that I was bad because I was doing them--I was a
bad person. That started a long time before--it
started in 5th grade so it had a really deep root that
I was a bad person. And when I tripped, it just opened
the doors--you're bad, no you're not, you're good,
you're good--and these conflicts would come out. It
would've been really good for me, I think if I could
have understood the feelings that I was getting when
I did acid. But I couldn't understand them at all,
I had no one to guide me. I was just lost in this infinite number of feelings and horrible things and good
things, just lost. I wish that I had had a guide or
someone that could have said, "Well, let's look at
those things that you're getting when you do acid, let's
see where they're coming from." But I couldn't look
at them. I was so confused I couldn't do anything
except go "aaah" and freak out.

A few weeks later she took some powerful acid at home, and
couldn't come down. Her psychiatrist, who she considers irrelevant and destructive to the process within her, hospitalized
her. She ran away from the hospital when she came down from
the trip, and moved first to a foster home, than a communal run-
away house, where she found the support she needed, and incidentally stopped using most drugs.

The alternative to hospital treatment is the growing numbers of free clinics, crisis centers and switchboards, where
young people who are experienced with psychedelics themselves,
help each other. Many hospitals refer psychedelic cases to
such groups, who deal with trips without fear and anxiety, and
with the understanding that the experience should be a positive
one. Such groups reflect the values of the counter culture, and
share the positive value on self exploration through psychedelics,
and through other growth experiences ranging from encounter
groups, meditation to art and service to others. Such centers
do not consider the process of investigating inner experience,
fantasy and feelings, understanding who one is or going deep
into oneself, as a cure for feelings of personal discomfort or
dissatisfaction with the world, or oneself. Crisis centers do
not aim at cures, or management of bad trips, but rather value
the process of exploration as an end in itself.

The process of intervention with a tripper starts when the
person enters. Rather than ask questions, the staff is able to

recognize what is happening, and someone with trip experience
takes the person to the area or room where the setting is peace-
ful, warm and comfortable, often like a womb as a conscious
attempt to legitimate regressive fantasies. The guide assures
the tripper that his feelings are all right, that he is on acid,
and that he should not fear his experience. It is often necessary to reassure the person that he is good, that his body is
good, that sex is good, that whatever he is guilty or in conflict about is a legitimate part of himself. Feelings are gone
into, by suggesting that the tripper go into them, and feel it as
much as he wants. If he is crying, he is told that he can cry
more if he wants, always reinforcing the validity of the feelings
being expressed, and being present like a parent, to comfort and
help the person, phsyically and emotionally, as long as necessary.
Such interventions take the duration of the trip, and some time
afterwards for working through, and there are no medical short-
cuts, unless the person is perfectly calm and says that he can be
left alone.

The guide is there to support the positive expression of
feelings, and to lessen the fear of the experience by reinforcing
the positive side of ambivalences. This usually helps the tripper resolve conflicts between wishes and fears, in favor of the
wish for expression. The guide supports, never by telling the
person what to do, and only to prevent destruction or physical
harm should the person be restrained. A good trip area is soft
and durable enough to allow restraint to be a minimum. When the
person comes down a working through session is the critical
point of the trip. Similar to a regular therapy session, the
guide talks to the tripper about what happened, so that the feelings which came up are not treated as foreign bodies which possessed him, but as valid and legitimate parts of himself. The
session goes over whatever painful but real feelings are still
unresolved. Memory of a trip is acute, but mechanisms of denial
and other defenses begin to operate immediately afterwards, and
if the followup sessions are not successful, all gain from the
trip will be lost.

The creation of crisis centers is the most feasible way for
young people to alleviate the potential harm which psychedelics
may do to them. The fact that young people are using drugs is
a given, and while social policies dream of control, independent
crisis centers are becoming increasingly valuable as way stations
for young people undergoing crisis which may or may not be related to drugs. The use of psychedelics by young people is a calculated risk by young people, which is healthy and adaptive behavior in the current conflict of values. As it becomes apparent
that psychedelics will not be controlled, suggestions like the
one voted down in Canada make more sense--that places be created
where people can have supervised psychedelic experiences.

Sara's Odyssey. This is a complete account of a psychedelic
intervention, written by Yvonne Jaffe, who was the guide. It
illustrates how even a completely negative set can be transformed
into a peak experience. It also illustrates the possibilities
for new styles of therapy, in this case regression as a way of
overcoming conflicts which block completely positive outcomes.
This is not a recommended procedure, but is rather a model for
what future life-transition crises can lead to.

Sara was almost 16, and needed space to grow. Her confused
feelings and contradictions burst the constricted boundaries of
her childhood self. She read about Che dying in her native land,
and about war and injustice in new adopted country, yet none of
this connected with her suburban existence. Her family related
to her as a child, awakening sexuality conflicted with Catholic
upbringing, and a neutral school experience all created feelings
of anger and frustration. These events were not talked about or
dealt with in her environment. She left one night.

When she arrived in New Haven she made her way to the green,
and struck up conversations, asking for friendship, help and
shelter. Sara's fears and doubts about herself were amplified
by the pressures of survival in marginal society, which were expressed to her as "a bed for a lay." The police-induced paranoia about informers had undermined the youth culture's desire
to be open and share, further hurting Sara's chances of making
contact. Eventually she was directed to Number Nine, the social
welfare and mental health arm of the new culture. She walked
into Nine, feeling things out, and eventually made her way up-
stairs to where counseling, crisis intervention and bad trip
help are offered. The rooms are curtained off, with old sofas
or mattresses covered with fabric, rug scraps on the floors, and
murals on the walls. She received shelter for a few days at
Nine's crash pad, and then moved into a new friend's apartment.
Sex brought her in contact with feelings she had defended against;
fear, guilt, loneliness and alarm at not having her parents nearby or finding a place where she felt safe. She was bombarded with
sensation she had no categories to deal with.

Sara felt like hurting herself. She had heard from drug
education classes that with LSD "you have all those bummers," so
she took a tab of acid. The fears she was holding back over-
whelmed her. She responded by regressing back to an earlier
stage of growth when she was more comfortable and secure, which
is a common defensive maneuver when psychedelics open the lid
too fast. She began to cry, moan and act afraid and upset. Her
friends took her back to Nine, for help. Most people on the
staff are personally familiar with LSD phenomena, and Sara's
acting out strong feelings with her whole body was instantly
recognized.

Sara's account of what she felt during her trip, which was
taped when she returned two weeks later, shows the importance of
the setting to transform an initial negative set.

> I was feeling very depressed, and I had tried to kill
> myself, so I thought I'd just become an acid head or
> speed freak or something. I expected it to be like
> going crazy and I was surprised it turned out so dif-
> ferently, because of the state of mind I was in. Maybe
> it was the surroundings. I'll never forget what hap-
> pened in that room, because it's been so important to
> me.

There were three distinct stages to her trip, and this progression is reported by Grof and others. The first stage encompasses the gradual *breaking down of her ego,* and a conflict
between guilt and fear, superego and id. Yvonne facilitated the
resolution of this conflict by creating a group fantasy with her,
embracing her, and finally having everyone take off their clothes
to increase her regression. That led to the second stage, a
death and rebirth. Sara wonders whether she deserves the pleasure she is having, and sees the guides as members of her family.
Her Oedipal conflict is resolved symbolically in the manner described by Norman O. Brown in *Love's Body,* not through identification with one parent but through union with both parents in and
through intercourse. The third stage follows quickly her death/
unification, and is the *peak experience.* She talks of white
light, starting a new world, milk, and takes on characteristics
of both man and woman, who she sees as unified. After the trip
came a difficult period of working through.

At first Sara huddled in the corner and cried out in Spanish,
her native language which she had not used regularly for years,
"Mike Samuels I love you. I need you. I want to die." Yvonne
was called in because she is Spanish also, and Jerry and Billy,
two other staff help. Sara repeated those phrases, which is a
common trip sign of a psychic conflict. The repetition is usually an internal dialogue between a wish (in this case for live,
closeness and sexual pleasure) and fears and guilt associated with
satisfying it (punishment by dying), which indicates that it is
not getting resolved. Yvonne encouraged her to express the feelings she blocked, and work through a fantasy solution, which will
then be vividly remembered as an experience which resolved the
conflict.

Sara was afraid and in need of support and security. She
was on such a regressed level that the most meaningful support
would be physical contact with a surrogate mother (of either sex).
Yvonne took this role, telling her not to be afraid and bathing
her hands and feet with a wet handkerchief. Yvonne saw her

withdraw slightly, and took this as a sign that she was working on negative feelings about touching her body. It is easy to build rapport with someone tripping, even when the guide and tripper have never met, because the tripper relates to people mainly as fantasy versions of parents and other important figures in their life.

Mothering is best when it is physical and direct. Words are confusing and often not understood, because the tripper may regress to a period before language. The integrity and self-awareness of the guide in this role is critical. He or she must move with the tripper, not seeking power or advantage over them, because people on psychedelics are unusually sensitive to this. The work of John Rosen (*Direct Psychoanalysis*), Margaret Seche-haye (*Autobiography of a Schizophrenic Girl*) and people who lived at Kingsley Hall (Laing, Joseph Berke and others) with psychosis support the contention that a mother-surrogate whose life is more unconditional than the original, can undo some of the damage in people who are much more fearful than Sara. The trip out of psychosis, while much longer, can be similar and demands the same kind of patience from the guide/mother.

Once contact is made, the guide can tune into the conflict the tripper is experiencing. There are only a small number of themes which make up the human condition, with infinite variations. Since they involve sexuality, guilt, union with parents, or desire for closeness and intimacy, the guide can test for the relevant theme by suggesting phrases which relate the tripper's words or actions to possible sources of the conflict, and judge from the reaction whether the trial is correct. If the theme suggested by the guide is not relevant, the tripper will simply ignore it, since LSD frees one almost totally from social games and polite conventions. Under acid all relationships relate directly to central needs.

Yvonne began this trial and error process from Sara's words. When Yvonne bathed her, Sara asked, "Lesbian?" Yvonne answered, "No, I'm not a lesbian, I'm Yvonne." This alerted Yvonne that while Sara might enjoy contact with a mother, this wish was in conflict with a fear that enjoying such contact was bad. Sara associated this fear with lesbianism as a defense against her desire for contact with women. Sara's contacts were soon resolved in favor of expression of positive feelings, as her words show:

> I remember Billy, he was my father, and Yvonne, she was my mother, and they were welcoming me from all the harships I had gone through. It was like a trial, and I kept asking them, "Am I deserving of all this pleasure?" I could feel all these tender feelings, as a

physical thing. I was free of all inhibitions, and
could hug them and do all the things...and I could,
and I did! I remember kissing my mother on the mouth,
which you know I was always told not to do. I really
wanted to hug and kiss her and even make love to her.
There was music and it was the Spanish setting, and
Yvonne had on a purple dress and long skirt, and
her breasts were coming out, and she was telling me,
"See, breasts are beautiful. You shouldn't be
ashamed of them." I wanted milk and I wanted love.
I told Yvonne I wanted to be breast-fed.

The infantile themes of union with mother and nourishment are inseparable from sexual themes. Sara told us later that for her
the *experience* (not the intellectual insight) of food and sex
were connected.

When Jerry came into the room, Yvonne asked if he was her
friend Mike, trying to incorporate him into the fantasy. Sara
said, "No, he's Jerry." Yvonne asked if she loved him, and she
said yes. Yvonne asked, "Would you like to fuck him?" tuning in
on the sexual implications of her impish grin. Such direct
language commonly is used in fantasies but rarely in unselfcon-
scious conversation. Yvonne talks that way to legitimate such
intimate sexual fantasy conversation. Sara at first embarras-
sedly tries to ignore the word, but then agrees that her need
for Mike Samuels is sexual. She says she wants Mike inside her,
but that this will cause her to die. She was given a phallic-
looking object to play with, which she alternately sucked and
moved between her legs.

Another common theme Sara was working through was rejection
of the body. Sara felt guilty about her previous sexual contact
with Mike, especially her enjoyment of physical intimacy. She
kept repeating, "Do I deserve it?" at every stage of her trip.
The guides reinforced her good feelings when she would smile and
say that sex is good, by replying that bodies were beautiful,
like a Greek chorus underscoring the message. Yvonne felt that
Sara would be still freer to express her sexuality and become
aware of her body as everyone took off their clothes. She expected Sara to follow suit, and that the sight of genitals would
focus some of her fantasies.

In the counter culture nudity is not especially unusual.
While this procedure may ignite fears of orgies and sexuality out
of control, even by prominent psychiatrists emerging from the
radical sexual tradition of Freud. Open expression of sexual
feelings and fantasies and baring the body is not particularly
dangerous, nor is it that helpful or revolutionary. For someone
like Sara, who has been taught to feel guilty around the very

existence of her body, the experience of social nakedness can
help her feel that there is nothing particularly dangerous, fearful or shameful about genitals. Nudity is actually experienced
as beautiful and natural, as growth centers like Esalen demonstrate, and Sara's account of her feelings during the trip bears
this out.

At first she pulled back in surprise and refused to look.
But she was obviously fascinated by the men's genitals, gradually
allowing her childish feelings of awe and curiosity to come out
on her face. Everybody hugged her, and chorused that bodies were
nice, and Sara agreed. She began to smile, at first guiltily
then more broadly, saying she didn't deserve it. The struggle
between opposing forces seemed to lessen, and her natural desire
to openly express her sexual feelings seemed to overcome guilt
and fear. Sara remembers the nudity as:

> sort of an Adam and Eve thing, it was so natural.
> I was so surprised at first because I knew I had all
> these inhibitions, like those parts of your body are
> not to be seen. I went to a nun's school and they
> really mess you up about that. I remember I wanted
> to get nude, in my life, in front of everybody. At
> first I was scared, and felt Yvonne was going to rape
> me, but then I knew that was what I really wanted.
> Like these ideas were always in back of my head, in
> my subconscious, but now I realized them. Of course
> I still have bad feelings about myself, but I feel
> now that I want to do something about it.

The dramatic action of the next part of her trip was Sara's
death and rebirth as part of a new culture. It is remarkable that
she sees symbolic connections which usually accompany only long-
term therapy, and does this without the interpretive mediation of
a therapist. Sara saw her death as a symbolic suicide caused by
her guilt about sex. But in this case the suicide was also revitalizing.

> I can remember that this guy I met, Mike Samuels, was
> in the room, and was saying things like "I only went
> out with her a couple of times." I was sort of hung
> up on him. I remember I was afraid to make love to
> him, and I'd like go frigid, and he told me, "You're
> so fucked up it makes me sick." every day I'd get up
> and think about that, and it was driving me crazy,
> it was all I'd think about.

When she kept repeating his name, the staff called him up, not
being sure of his relationship to her. He came down, but was
obviously too anxious about the incident himself, that he stayed

only a minute, long enough for Sara to hug him and ask him to make love to her, and then spent the evening talking to Dennis about his own confusions.

Sara's account continues:

So when I died, I remember calling him on a street corner, all hunched up and there were people around me, saying that I was gonna die now. First they took me to an institution, because I had gone made or something. That was here, Number Nine. And I was saying I was crazy in Spanish, I went through a lot and I had to die in order to be reborn again. My heartbeat started to get slower and slower. I remember I'm going to die, there's no place to go, it's going to be like when I was born, nothing, and I don't want it to be like that. I wanted to be something, not nothingness.

Many of these themes take on additional meaning when compared to Buddhist or Tibetan texts, which are guides for people undergoing such experiences in their natural deaths.

When I was born again it was like paradise, it was so beautiful! It's like I came through this light, but they expected it and I expected it. I could hear an ambulance, and it was like they were bringing me. It was my mother, and I'm coming out to her, and I did. Everybody was there to see it, and everybody's eyes were tearful with the joy. It was like utopia, I felt feelings that were indescribable. There was happiness and joy and I was crying. I was born with everything, all this knowledge. I remember the press or something was there and they were going to print it. It was our world, maybe the whole world had died off and we were the new culture. My parents were there and I wanted to be part of them both, to make love to both of them, like I had to have their approval because I was part of them. There was little colored twinkling things all around, and it was like we had made this world, because we were so strong. I remember we were going out to cut cane, and our hands were so calloused. I remember putting these boots on, and Yvonne telling me, "But darling, put these clothes on because tomorrow is another day, and we're going to start." Now I remember I didn't want to go to sleep, because I wanted to start right now having babies and working for the new culture.

A later theme was the idealization of her father and masculinity,

and the realization that male qualities existed in her. She saw
the conflicting elements, like maleness and femaleness, yin and
yang, childishness and adulthood, not in conflict, but existing
simultaneously within her.

> It was this brotherhood feeling and everyone was shar-
> ing it. Billy was sitting in the chair. He was like
> one of those Indian gurus also, and I was saying,
> "Daddy, I want to make love to you, I don't want to
> wait any more." He said that I had to. Then we were
> going out to cut cane, and he was Che Guevara, and he
> was my father. I kept thinking about the milk and
> Yvonne, and then I remember smoking a cigar, and I
> was Che. I was both a man and a woman. That was the
> most beautiful thing. I could be both. I could be
> gentle and the maternal type of thing, and I could
> also be strong and lead. I remember I was with my
> family, and there were three guys, brothers or some-
> thing, and I had to choose between them. I think it
> was Jerry who was like the sweetness, the tender type
> of part, the shy part. And then Billy, he was the
> revolutionary type, and then somebody else, Dennis,
> represented wisdom and knowledge and everything. Then
> they told me that you have to choose which of your
> parents you want, and I told them, "No, I can have
> both." And I was so happy, and it was so beautiful.

Towards the end everyone helped Sara relax with massage.
She talked about what she wants to do in her life, of school,
writing, and making the world a better place to live. She
stayed at Nine, and tried to make love to everyone, but was
gently put off. She was helped to take a shower and then fell
asleep. The next day Yvonne woke her, and found her depressed
and guilt-ridden. Yvonne reviewed the trip, explaining that
those feelings were real, and she should accept them as part of
her. Sara refused to talk, and said finally she wanted to see
it as a dream, because she saw now that was not the way things
are. She left soon after. When she came back two weeks later,
she was beaming and smiling, wearing colorful clothes and a
bright rainbow shawl. She thanked us for the experience, and
her face was as radiant as it had been during the trip, in sharp
contrast to the subdued demeanor before and immediately after it.
Her account validated our impression of the significance of the
trip, and how much she had uncovered and learned to accept about
herself.

She ends her narrative with her conclusions:

> Right after the trip I didn't really know what I had
> done, but I felt guilty anyway. When I woke up it was

so different. Then I started reconstructing things,
and I realized it was true, that's your subconscious
and that's how you feel. I started feeling that we
really have to live to satisfy ourselves. Not be
selfish you know, but you can't satisfy anyone if
you're not satisfied yourself. That's my main goal
now. Before I was so afraid of being hurt that I
built this wall and made myself a prisoner in it. I've
changed now. Like before I'd just sit in a corner and
sulk, and if somebody talked to me I wouldn't even
talk to them. I'd just nod. My feelings have been
blocked and sterile. I couldn't communicate with
people. Like I wanted to shout "I love you" or "I
just want to hold your hand" or something like that,
but I couldn't because I was so restrained. We have
only one of those things we call lives, and we breathe
and walk around and things like that, and poof, it's
gone. As far as I'm concerned there's nothing else,
as far as positive proof is concerned, so I'd better
make sure I make something of it, enjoy myself.

The trip intervention turned what was intended as an act
of self-destruction into an opening-up peak experience. Because
other tremendous insight and capacity to integrate learning,
Sara has been freed up since then to trust people more and express herself without drugs, and she has no desire to trip again.
Through counseling and group experience at Number Nine, she continues to relate her insights to her everyday life. She contacted her parents, and talked about what she is doing and some
of the feelings she was holding back. She visited home, and
her family agreed that she could continue to live in New Haven,
in a residential job corps program.

Transitional Communities. Both psychedelic drugs and the
support community which helped Sara play critical roles in the
development of a new culture. The themes and visions which came
to Sara while tripping are a spontaneous personal rediscovery of
the central values of the counter culture. Psychedelics seem
to have catalyzed a vision of what can be, and release enough
dammed up energy to lead many to actualize these values in their
non-drug experiences. The convergence in Sara's trip of Maslow's
Being values and the themes of the counter culture lead to speculation about whether this new culture, born of drugs, may have
recovered some bedrock truths about the deepest levels of the
psyche, which the dominant culture has lost sight of. This is
the thesis of Maslow, psychedelic researchers and youth. Sara's
story shows some of the fruits of young people's exploration of
the deeper levels of their psyche. The new culture holds the
possibility of a nonrepressive culture, which can be developed
through communal living, encounter groups, sexual exploration,

the study of other cultures and religions, and the restructuring
of political institutions.

Sara's journey also demonstrates how the developmental
crisis which are exposed by drug use can be worked through constructively, without psychic damage or the destructive effects
of an exploitive environment. With the recognition that our
culture is in a new form of transition, the Protean Man which
Robert Lifton describes, provisions should be made so that risks
of young people in drugs and new communities do not lead to harm.
Alvin Toffler, in *Future-Shock*, suggests that we need transition
communities to help us cope with the onslaught of rapid change.
Growing up and changing is now a lifetime job. As an adaptive
strategy, the experimentation that young people choose through
psychedelics and new communities is a healthy survival mechanism.
Adaptation is the way to survival during change. The most rapid
changes take place in the young, who bring new energy and flexibility to a totally new and threatening situation. Education
is antithetical to these changes, as it disallows feelings and
experiment and promotes conformity to an authority which no
longer makes sense. They must go out and seek learning by taking
risks and developing learning opportunities. They use psychedelics as one form of antidote to their education and environment,
as a way of breaking up patterns and enabling them to create new
ones. Communities like Number Nine can develop into the new
learning centers, as well as spaces to work through personal
crisis on the way.

In a time of confusion, conflict and cultureal transition,
the best that people can do is search together for answers and
possibilities that do not yet exist. The future of any new culture lies with transition communities which can be formed to support and focus growing attempts at self-definition. New learning tools like psychedelic drugs are being harnessed to help
people grow, despite the persecution of drug users by the dominant culture. Their controls have no teeth, so exploration goes
on, albeit with frustration and occasional harassment. Only a
world-view which emphasizes change, risk openness to inner experience and exploration can cope with our changing environment.
A psychology which emphasizes sickness, man's evil, caution and
self-control is outmoded and self-defeating. People like Sara
should not be adjusted or controlled by the dominant culture
which she does not want. She must be free to grow beyond it.

NOTE: An altered version of this chapter appears in Chapter 4
*Toward a Radical Therapy: Alternate Services for Personal and
Social Change* by Clark, T. and Jaffe, D., published by Gordon
and Breach, 1973.

REFERENCES

Blewett, D. *Frontiers of being.* New York: Award Paperback, 1969.

Cohen, S. Lysergic Acid Diethlyamide: Side effects and complications. *Journal of Nervous and Mental Disease,* 1960, *130,* 30-40.

Erikson, K. T. *Wayward puritans.* New York: Wiley, 1966.

Grof, S. *Theory and practice of LSD psychotherapy.* State College: University of Pennsylvania Press, 1973.

Harman, W. The issue of consciousness-expanding drug. *Main Currents of Modern Thought.* Vol. 20, *1,* 1963.

Laing, R. D. *Politics of experience.* New York: Pantheon, 1967.

Laing, R. D. *Knots.* New York: Pantheon, 1971.

Laing, R. D. *Politics of the family.* New York: Pantheon, 1971.

Lifton, R. J. *Boundaries: Psychological man in revolution.* New York: Random House, 1970.

Maslow, A. *Toward a psychology of being.* New York: Von Nostrand, 1968.

Pahnke, W., Kurland, A., Unger, S., Savage, C. & Grof, S.   The experimental use of psychedelic (LSD) psychotherapy. *Journal of the American Medical Association,* June 15, 1970, *212,* 1856-1863.

Rosen, J. N. *Direct analysis: Selected papers.* New York: Grune and Stratton, 1953.

Savage, C. & Stolaroff, M. Clarifying the confusion regarding LSD-25. *Journal of Nervous and Mental Disease.* 1965, *140,* 218-221.

Slater, P. E. *Pursuit of loneliness.* Boston: Beacon, 1971.

Sechehaye, M. *Autobiography of a schizophrenic girl.* Translated by Grace Rubin-Rabson. New York: New American Library, 1970.

Szasz, T. S. *Manufacture of madness.* Scranton, Pa.: Harper and Row, 1970.

Taylor, R., Maurer, J. & Tinklenberg, J. Management of "Bad Trips" in an evolving drug scene. *Journal of the American Medical Association,* July 20, 1970, *213,* 422-425.

Toffler, A. *Future shock.* New York: Random House, 1970.

Van Dusen, W. LSD and the enlightenment of Zen. *Psychologia,* 1961, *4* .

12:   FAMILY CRISIS THERAPY

In this chapter, Goldstein and Giddings describe the rationale and proposed procedure for working with families in crisis. Their work represents an extention of an interventive model developed for adolescents and their families into the realm of families with young children. The basic argument presented for the approach involves the conceptualization of the family group as being functionally analogous to the individual. Like an individual, a family can find its coping resources overtaxed, succumb to disorganization, readapt around emergency coping strategies and grow or suffer as a consequence of the new solutions. Goldstein and Giddings further assert that periods of family crisis, like periods of personal crisis, increase the likelihood that outside intervention will be accepted and effectively utilized.

The specific interventive approach initially requires a sophisticated assessment of the family's potential for being helped, prior to intensive but very short term intervention where indicated. This approach, labeled "multiple impact therapy" (MIT) is described as a realtively structured program requiring only one day of intense antivity. Family members are to be in individual, joint and overlapping sessions conducted by a team of workers. Data on the instantaneous state of family relations is collected periodically throughout the treatment day, both to guide the team and to study the technique. Thus, as in the work of Freitag, Goldstein and Giddings outline a program of service integrated with research.

The intervention described in this chapter is not to be the work of untrained or minimally trained personnel. Goldstein and Giddings are suggesting a treatment model which clearly requires the direct services of mental health professionals. The extreme brevity of the treatment, however, allows for the possibility that the program would not require the profligate use of manpower resources.

Unlike most programs of family intervention, this proposal based on a crisis model does not stipulate a goal of raising the family to new heights of interpersonal functioning, but rather aims at restoring the family to the pre-crisis level where earlier coping mechanisms will again function effectively. Given the lack of actual data, one may only speculate about the efficacy of the approach. One interesting question is whether this mode of treatment, which requires a consensual family commitment to an intense unfamiliar experience, will actually be accepted by families that could benefit. Another issue which might be considered in evaluating the proposed intervention is whether young children could handle the fast pace and potentially high anxiety of the treatment day. The authors do not specify what strategy would be employed if a child, or other family member, refuses to persevere in the treatment or becomes too upset to continue.

MULTIPLE IMPACT THERAPY:

AN APPROACH TO CRISIS INTERVENTION WITH FAMILIES

Sondra Goldstein and John Giddings

Pittsburgh Child Guidance Center

Crisis has been broadly defined by Gerald Caplan as an "upset in a steady state" (Caplan, 1964). According to concept of crisis developed by Caplan, Lindemann, Klein, *et al.* (1961) a family is usually in a state of relative equilibrium maintained by complicated interchanges among family members. This "steady state" is particularly dependent upon the interpersonal transactions through which individual family members gratify their emotional needs. Occasions arise, however, when a family is incapable of solving problems that have been brought about by hazardous circumstances, and the usual homeostatic mechanisms are unsuccessful in restoring the previous equilibrium. A more or less protracted period of emotional upset follows that is called a crisis.

Caplan (1964) states that the most common "hazardous circumstances" which may precipitate crises are biological or role transitions: birth, puberty, climacteric, illness or death, entry into kindergarten, transfer to grade school, transfer to high school, leaving school, getting the first job. moving to a new community, getting a new job, undertaking new social or occupational responsibilities, or relinquishing job responsibility through retirement. Such circumstances constitute either a loss or threat of loss of basic supplies, or a challenge involving the possibility of greater supplies, but at a greater cost.

All families experience various "hazardous circumstances" yet not all families experience these events as crises. Hill (1965) points out that these events become crises according to the definition the family makes of the event. He gives the following formula for a crisis: A. (the event) interacting with B. (the family's crisis-meeting resources) interacting with C. (the definition the family gives the event) produces X. (the Crisis).

A crisis-proof family must have agreement in its role structure, satisfaction of the physical and emotional needs of its
members, and goals toward which the family is moving collectively. Having all of these, the family is adequately organized and has crisis-meeting resources. Lacking them, the family is inadequately organized, and likely to prove vulnerable
to crisis precipitating events. If a family has deficiencies
in crisis-meeting resources, they will tend to experience and
define hazardous circumstances as crises.

After an inadequately organized family has defined an
event as a crisis, there follows a period during which solutions
to the crisis are worked out. During this time certain patterns
may evolve in which tension is reduced for the family as a group,
but at the emotional expense of one or more family members.
This can happen in two ways: passively, by emotional neglect,
i.e., concentrating family energies such that the needs of an
individual are not attended; and actively, by the emotional exploitation of a family member, *i.e.*, investing him with a role
that does violence to his individual needs. This mechanism reduces group tension by allowing displacement of individual anxieties or ventilation of guilt in relation to the scapegoated
individual (Parad & Caplan, 1965). Typically the scapegoated
person then bears the burden of, and acts out the family's tension and anxiety. This pattern of crisis resolution is often
found in families where one member is a disturbed child or
adolescent.

Periods of equilibrium may occur following crisis-resolution at the expense of an individual family member. However,
as new hazardous circumstances occur, the usual solution of
scapegoating may be made less available to the family. For
example, the school may begin to complain about a disturbed
child's behavior, or an adolescent may rebel against his role
as a scapegoat. When the usual crisis-resolution pattern is
not available or effective for the family, there is an increase
in tension and a state of upset and ineffectuality. The feelings of helplessness engendered by this state may prompt a family to seek help outside the family orbit. The aid of relatives, friends, police, school officials, physicians, etc. may
be sought.

Another frequent alternative is family referral of the disturbed child or adolescent to a treatment center. On one level,
this is yet another attempt by the family at crisis resolution
via scapegoating of one member. However, if this solution were
effectively functioning for the family, there would be no referral of the child. Thus, the referral itself indicates that the
family is experiencing tension and disequilibrium, and is seeking a novel solution to its crisis.

Many authors (Waldfogel & Gardner, 1961; Rapaport, 1965; Kauffman, 1965) view the family in crisis as more susceptible to the influence of "significant others" in the environment. Klein and Lindemann (1961) state that in working with a family in crisis a maximum of change may be possible with a minimum of effort. Caplan (1961) asserts that families in crisis can be put back onto a healthy path, and this can be done without having to analyze the "original deep reasons inside the personalities of these people which made it difficult for them to handle the problem in a healthy way." Thus, a little help, rationally directed and purposefully focused at a strategic time, may be more effective than more extensive help given at a period of less emotional accessibility. A state of crisis has growth promoting potential in that it may act as a catalyst to disrupt old habits and evoke new responses. A crisis may bring forth new coping mechanisms which serve to strengthen the family's adaptive capacity and thereby raise the family's general level of mental health.

Short-term crisis intervention techniques have been found effective in dealing with a variety of family problems. Thompson and Wiley (1970) developed a short-term group approach utilizing crisis-intervention principles for families of hospitalized mental patients. Tooley (1970) modified pathological family reactions to moving by limited-goal, brief psychotherapy. Langsley *et al.* (1968a) found that family crisis therapy was effective in keeping disturbed family members from hospitalization. Langsley *et al.* (1968b) found a family crisis therapy approach effective in reducing family tensions brought about by an acting-out adolescent. Shaw *et al.* (1968) found that short term therapy (12 sessions) including individual, parent, and family interviews, was particularly effective in dealing with school phobia and inhibition of aggression in children. Duckworth (1967) found crisis focused therapy effective for a wide range of family difficulties, *e.g.*, anxiety reactions, school phobia, mental breakdown, delinquency, and situational stresses. The latter approach appeared to reach more low-socioeconomic clients, and to resolve problems in less time (6-8 weeks) than usual methods.

MacGregor *et al.* (1965) developed the multiple impact therapy (MIT) approach for disturbed adolescents and families. MIT is a brief, usually two-day, intensive study and treatment of a family in crisis. The approach is based on two assumptions. First, individuals and families facing a crisis are stimulated to mobilize strength and resources to meet it, and they are more receptive to interpretations, more likely to be flexible in attitude, than at other times. The second assumption is that in any type of psychotherapy, there is likely to be faster and more dramatic change in the early stages of treatment, and that

under longer-term treatment, later change and development is
more gradual, is a deepening and strengthening of the initial
movement during the first hours or weeks, toward improved
health or adjustment.

The procedures developed by MacGregor *et al.* (1965) con-
sisted essentially of an initial family team conference, followed by a series of individual interviews, joint interviews
(two patients with one or more therapists, or two therapists
with one or more patients), and overlapping interviews (therapist terminates his interview with one family member and joins
another in conference, either alone or accompanied by the person he has been seeing). Psychological tests are given to the
adolescent during the first afternoon, and results are shared
in a general way with the parents and adolescent, usually early
the second day. The two-day contact terminates with a final
family-team conference, and in this last conference the "back
home" problem is discussed in terms of specific recommendations,
and insights gained during the preceding day and a half are
applied to behavior and situations that can be anticipated. A
follow-up conference six months later is arranged, primarily
for the benefit of the research team, to evaluate the results
of MIT with the family.

MacGregor *et al.* have utilized MIT for treatment of a wide
range of presenting problems and types of crises. These included chronic runaways, delinquent acting-out behaviors, school
failure, school phobia, sexual deviations, with a range of diagnostic categories from adjustment reactions through the schizo-
phrenias. The authors state that MIT is the method of choice
for initiating therapy when a family crisis exists; it is also
the method of choice for creating a salutary crisis within a
family in treatment where an intrafamilial stalemate exists.

To evaluate the effectiveness of the MIT approach, Mac-
Gregor *et al.* obtained follow-up information on 62 families at
six and eighteen month intervals following the initial MIT procedures. The team rated the nominal patient on seven categories, *e.g.*, relationship with age mates, sex role in relation
to parents, attitude toward authority, etc., and also rated
intrafamilial patterns using ten categories, *e.g.*, sibling situation, patterns of fatherhood, patterns of motherhood, family
response to crises, etc.

Results of ratings of the 62 families showed a favorable
outcome of 49 cases, and unfavorable outcome of 13 cases. The
type of movement noted in all favorable outcomes was generally
in the hypothesized direction of movement from stereotyped balance of power family relations, which induced arrest in development by forcing each family member to continue excessively in a

single role, to a more flexible interaction that allowed growth changes for all members.

Although MIT was originally developed for use with adolescents and their families, the approach appears to be equally applicable to families in which the crisis centers around a child. In order to assess the usefulness of an MIT approach with a child guidance population, an MIT treatment and research pilot project is presently being developed at the Pittsburgh Child Guidance Center. Interdisciplinary teams are participating in the pilot project utilizing a modified MIT plan similar to the plan developed by MacGregor *et al.* (1965). MIT will be available as the treatment of choice when a family crisis exists; it will also be available for creating a salutary crisis within a family engaged in traditional treatment where an intrafamilial stalemate exists.

The MIT procedures are quite flexible, but are usually a one-and-one-half hour intake session with the entire family and team, followed by a one-day intensive treatment of the family by the guidance clinic team.

In the intake conference the family is invited to explain the problem of crisis to the team. Usually one family will act as spokesman initially; the team then encourages participation from the others. All questions and comments to encourage participation are worded to convey respect for feelings and opinions of each family member, and to convey the team's recognition that the behavior of each must have "made sense" at the time if viewed in terms of the situation. Interpretations and even speculation are begun by the team in the intake session. A tentative formulation and re-statement of the family problems is made by the team at the end of the intake conference. A contract with the family is then made for the one-day MIT.

The one-day intensive treatment consists of an initial team-family conference, followed by a series of individual, joint, and overlapping interviews. The day terminates with a final family-team conference at which the referral problem or crisis is discussed in terms of insights gained during the day of treatment. Specific recommendations are made in the final conference about applications of insight to behavior and situations that can be anticipated. In some cases recommendations may include a second day of MIT, or continuation of the family in treatment already begun.

All families will be evaluated prior to MIT treatment, and at a one month interval following the MIT day. A discussion of the treatment and research techniques to be used in the MIT pilot project follows.

METHOD

Referral

The first step in this approach occurs when a given family
is referred to the MIT team. This group, including child psychiatrists, clinical psychologists, and social workers, reviews
the available material on the family and decides whether the
family should be invited to the center for an intake session.
The decision at this point will be based upon the presence of
a family crisis that the family seems unable to meet. The team
will analyze the available material for evidence that there is
disagreement within the family role structure, a lack of satisfaction of emotional needs, an absence of goals towards which
the family is moving collectively, and inadequate coping mechanisms. The team will also base its decision upon the likelihood
of benefits of an intensive therapeutic approach. If the criteria are met, then one of the team members contacts the family
by phone and invites them to the center for an intake session.

Intake

When the family arrives at the center, they will be met by
the team member who has had contact with the family. They will
be taken to the primary treatment room where the other members
of the treatment team are waiting. This room is large enough
to accommodate most families and has a one way mirror which permits audio and video recording as well as observation of the
multiple impact therapy. At the beginning of the intake session
the family will be told that audio and video recordings will be
made of all sessions with them for research and training purposes.

When the family arrives at the treatment room, the first
phase of the session will allow the family to meet the treatment team and become more relaxed in this situation. If all
members of the family do not appear for the intake session,
inquiry is undertaken to determine the reasons for their absence. Next the family will be asked about the problems which
prompted them to seek help. Everyone in the family will be encouraged to present their views of the family problems.

After thirty minutes have elapsed, this discussion will be
interrupted and each family member will be asked to complete a
questionnaire examining the structure, strengths and weaknesses
of the family. Although the family members will be available

to provide assistance to the younger children, *e.g.*, if a child cannot write, a team member will write his answers for him. The family will be given twenty minutes to answer the questionnaire, after which the questionnaires will be collected even though they may not be complete. Next the family will be asked to discuss these questions for twenty minutes, and arrives at concensus answers. The team members will leave the room while the family arrives at their answers. This discussion and comparable discussions during the treatment and follow-up phases provide the data for the subsequent analyses of the effects of the MIT approach.

As the family discusses the questionnaire, they will be observed by the MIT team through the one way mirror. At this time the team will share impressions of the family dynamics, and reach a decision about the "suitability" of the MIT approach for the family. If the MIT approach seems appropriate for the family, the primary objective for the remainder of the intake session will be to establish a contract with the family to engage in the treatment day.

After twenty minutes have elapsed, the MIT team will return to the treatment room and collect the family questionnaire. The family will then be encouraged to discuss their problems further, including a description of their efforts to resolve these problems themselves. Following this discussion the team will present its observations of the family and its problems which suggest using the MIT approach. A specific proposal will be made inviting the family to spend a day with the MIT team to work on the family problems. If the family accepts this invitation, a specific date is set at that time.

Treatment Procedures

Although a general format has been developed for the MIT day, specific plans will be made for each family. Between the intake session and the MIT day, the team will review video and audio tapes of the intake session in order to further define the family dynamics and plan the treatment day. Each team member shares his impressions of the family and gives his formulation of the family difficulties. The team then plans the morning of the treatment day in terms of the therapist assignments to individual members and scheduling of joint and overlapping activities.

On the day set aside for this approach the family will be expected at the center at 9:00 a.m. The initial team-family conference will be held in the primary treatment room. Following a brief "social period" to allow the family to become more at ease in this setting, the team will initiate a one-hour discussion about events within the family since the intake session. The team will attempt to guide this discussion toward elaboration of the family's central problems.

Following the hour discussion the team will move to the center of the room, and will ask the family to observe and listen to them as they discuss their observations about the problems and rule of the family. This will allow the family to observe and be exposed to information about itself. During this discussion the team will also confirm or modify plans for the next phase of treatment, $i.e.$, individual, joint, and overlapping interviews. At the conclusion of the staff discussion, team members will move back to their original places in the circle, and encourage the family to express their reactions to the team's observations of the family.

The next phase of treatment (individual, joint, and overlapping interviews) is expected to last one hour. Then the team and family will come together and share what has taken place in these sessions. When this half-hour discussion is completed, the family will be asked to rejoin the team at 1:00 p.m. following a break for lunch.

The MIT team will have lunch together and plan the goals and strategies for the afternoon. The specific plans will depend upon the family difficulties, and upon what has occurred during the morning sessions. In general, the afternoon sessions will involve a joint team-family meeting, followed again by individual, joint and overlapping interviews.

The last segment of the day will provide an opportunity to summarize that which has taken place during the day, as well as permit the family to express their reactions to the MIT experience. The problems presented by the family are discussed in terms of specific recommendations and insights gained during the day. As the team summarizes and makes recommendations, the family will be encouraged to verbalize any remaining concerns and anticipated problems. The team will then encourage the family to try and handle these anticipated crises using the recommendations made during the MIT day.

The final thirty minutes of the day will be used to complete the tasks that were used in the intake session. Again each family member will be asked to complete the questionnaire individually. If necessary, assistance will be provided to younger children for this task. When fifteen minutes have passed, the individual questionnaires will be collected, and the family will be asked to complete the questionnaire together without the team members present. This discussion will provide the data for the second segment of family interaction.

Follow-up.

One month after the MIT day, the family will come to the center for a follow-up session. The purpose of this session will be to provide the MIT team an opportunity to evaluate the impact of the MIT procedures on the family. This session will include a discussion of the events within the family since the MIT day with emphasis upon the status of previously reported family problems and their current successes in coping with these problems.

Following this discussion each member of the family will be asked to complete the family questionnaire. Again, following individual questionnaire completion, the family will be asked to jointly work out answers to the questionnaire. The resulting family discussion will provide data for the final measure of family interaction.

EVALUATION OF THE MIT APPROACH

Three procedures will be employed to evaluate the impact of the MIT approach on the families in this study. The first procedure will be based upon an examination of the individual and family responses to the questionnaire. It will be possible to see if changes take place within individual family members' perceptions of family strengths, problems, and authority patterns. In addition, it will be possible to determine the extent to which there is agreement between the members of the family in their perceptions of the family. One can also examine the extent to which the presenting problems are seen as changing, or lessening from the beginning of intake to the end of treatment.

The second analysis will be based upon an examination of the ways the family has attempted to cope with their problems at the time of the intake session in comparison with their attempts to deal with their problems at the follow-up session.

The results of these two analyses should provide evidence about the effectiveness of the MIT approach in helping families in crisis become better able to cope with such crises, and in helping families experiencing an intrafamilial stalemate function in a less stereotyped manner. Further understanding of the impact of the MIT approach will be derived from the third research procedure to be employed in this study.

The third procedure will be an analysis of the family interaction patterns as they discuss the questionnaires by means
of Riskin's Family Interaction Scales (Riskin & Faunce, 1970),
a well researched method for studying family interaction patterns. The Interaction Scales provide meaningful and objective
measures of the family interaction, with six main categories of
family patterns:

(1) Clarity: whether the family members speak clearly to
one another; (2) Topic Continuity: whether family members stay
on the same topic with one another and when they shift topics;
(3) Commitment: whether the family members take direct stands
on issues and feelings with one another; (4) Agreement and
Disagreement: whether family members explicitly agree or dis-
agree with one another; (5) Affective Intensity, whether family
members show variations in affect as they communicate with one
another; and (6) Relationship Quality: whether family members
are friendly or attacking with one another. Riskin has demonstrated the reliability of these scales, and provides some evidence of the validity of certain scales with normal and problem
families. He suggests that the Interaction Scales might be useful in evaluating changes within families as a result of therapeutic intervention, but the scales have not been used to date
for this purpose.

In the present study the family discussion of the questionnaires will be analyzed using the Family Interaction Scales at
three different points: intake, at the end of the treatment day,
and in the follow-up session. The benefits of this analysis of
family interaction patterns should include additional information about the effectiveness of the MIT procedures with families
in crisis, and also the suitability of the Family Interaction
Scales for evaluating changes following family treatment.

REFERENCES

Caplan, G. *An approach to community mental health*. London: Tavistock Publications, 1961.

Caplan, G. *Principles of preventive psychiatry*. New York: Basic Books, Inc., 1964.

Duckworth, G. L. A project in crisis intervention. *Social Casework*, 1967, *48*, 227-31.

Faunce, E. E. & Riskin, J. Family interaction scales: II. Data analysis and findings. *Archives of General Psychiatry*, 1970, *22*, 513-526.

Hill, R. Generic features of families under stress. In H. J. Parad, (Ed.), *Crisis intervention: Selected readings*. New York: Family Service Association, 1965.

Kaffman, M. Short-term family therapy. In H. J. Parad (Ed.), *Crisis intervention: Selected readings*. New York: Family Service Association, 1965.

Klein, D. C. & Lindemann, E. Preventive intervention in individual and family crisis situations. In G. Caplan (Ed.), *Prevention of mental disorders in children*. New York: Basic Books, Inc., 1961.

Langsley, D. G., Pittman, F. S., Machatka, P., & Flomenhoft, K. Family crisis therapy: results and implications. *Family process*, 1968, *7*, 145-58.

Langsley, D. G., Fairbairn, R. H., & DeYoung, C. Adolescence and family crises. *Canadian Psychiatric Association Journal*, 1968, *13*, 125-33.

MacGregor, R., Ritchie, A. M., Serrano, A. C., & Schuster, F. P. *Multiple impact therapy with families*. New York: McGraw-Hill, 1964.

Parad, H. J., & Caplan, G. A framework for studying families in crisis. In H. J. Parad (Ed.), *Crisis intervention: Selected readings*. New York: Family Service Association, 1965.

Rapaport, R. Normal crises, family structure, and mental health. In H. J. Parad (Ed.), *Crisis intervention: Selected readings*. New York: Family Service Association, 1965.

Riskin, J., & Faunce, E.E. Family interaction scales: I. Theoretical framework and method. *Archives of General Psychiatry*, 1970, *22*, 504-12.

Riskin, J., & Faunce, E.E. Family interaction scales: III. Discussion of methodology and substantive findings. *Archives of General Psychiatry*, 1970, *22*, 527-37.

Shaw, R., Blumenfeld, H., & Senf, R. A short-term treatment program in a child guidance clinic. *Social work*, 1968, *13*, 81-90.

Thompson, R. W., & Wiley, E. Reaching families of hospitalized mental patients: a group approach. *Community Mental Health Journal*, 1970, *6*, 22-30.

Tooley, K. The role of geographic mobility in some adjustment problems of children and families. *Journal of the American Academy of Child Psychiatry*, 1970, *9*, 366-78.

Waldfogel, S., & Gardner, G. E. Intervention in crisis as a method of primary prevention. In G. Caplan (Ed.), *Prevention of mental disorders in children*. New York: Basic Books, Inc., 1961.

V: COMMENTS

The selections in this book provide, by example, a definition of the current crisis intervention domain. The chapters
present a diversity of perspectives and were written by people
of differing professional allegiance. In the following para-
graphs, some of the issues raised by our contributors are reviewed.

Unfortunately, as with many important mental health services, research and empirical support for crisis intervention
practice is limited. As can be gleaned from the chapters by
Stern and Bleach, research efforts are often resisted and, beyond the clinical anecdote, little knowledge of the effects of
crisis intervention practice has been accumulated. This situation seems to stem from two principle sources: the important
questions have not been asked, and most readily available methodologies are inadequate to the job.

Research in mental health practice has too often concentrated on the wrong questions, the answers to which do not have
an impact on field technique. For crisis intervention important
questions include: Who are the people receiving the crisis services? What are the characteristics of the crisis? What exis-
tent community resources for crisis intervention can be strength-
ened to improve service delivery? Are there identifiable groups
of people for whom the present form of crisis delivery is inappropriate or unavailable? Are there certain teachable techniques
which are known to be effective in ameliorating certain kinds of
crises? Which ones work in what context? What are the key
signs required for accurate selection of an appropriate crisis
intervention technique? Who should (or can) be trained, and how?

Clinical practice in crisis intervention is sustained, not
by logical positivist empiricism, but by personal feelings of
comfort, competence and professional role expectations. Several
authors argue that the crisis intervenor should be prepared to
give up his traditional "helping" role for a new ones featuring

less structure, fewer limitations and protections, and greater intrusion into the worker's private life. The Stern and Mc-Colskey chapters give evidence that these "new" roles can become constricted by tradition, rules of practice and policy. Only the Jaffe chapter indicates a dramatically different role for a crisis worker, and one which probably will be rejected by many readers. It is reasonable, however, to expect that within the "Number Nine" type of service agency, there also are defined limits of appropriate intervention. Role conflicts are an inevitable consequence of changing forms of service delivery.

One reason that traditional mental health services have had difficulty in responding quickly and effectively to the call for crisis intervention, is that most mental health training is strikingly unsuited to the responsiveness called for in the management of immediate crisis. Shneidman must remind us that dependency is not synonymous with pathology, Sebolt tells us of the unique role changes to expect, Levy shows us that the medical model does not generate appropriate responses to crisis, and Berman gives us examples of training which are far from the analyst's couch. However, our prejudices run deep; who among us would be willing to take off our clothes when working with a person in a drug crisis?

Freitag, *et al.*, Williams, and Goldstein & Giddings provide more traditional role responses to crisis intervention within the framework of a professional model. In the first case, professionals supervise the work of college students in the management of the hospital-to-home crisis for mental patients. William's program exemplifies the use of professionals to expand services by providing skills to naturally occurring help givers; however, the training suggested is within the traditional mold and does not call, as Jaffe would have us do, upon the unique features of the indigenous agent. The Goldstein and Giddings approach can be described as one which moves a service agency into dramatic action in order to have a radical impact on a family in crisis. This plan is consistent with that advocated by Shneidman, Korner and Sebolt, it represents, within traditional mental health service delivery, a potential source of agency change which produces an immediate impact on a client in crisis rather than a continuing routine of prolonged, extended, never resolved crisis. But even this plan consumes significant professional time and operates under the constraints of scheduling, location and staff involvement.

Albee and others have indicated that manpower needs within the traditional therapeutic model will never be met by the training systems now extant. Similarly, community resources are not likely to support endless professionals serving small numbers of clients for indeterminable periods. Several authors have suggested, either directly or indirectly, that the democratization of crisis service is a partial solution. Democratization in this case refers to the provision of services to more clients by more people devoid of strong guild, hierarchy, or status loyalties. While McColskey, Korner and Goldstein & Giddings could be interpreted as advocating sophisticated clinical training for crisis workers and retaining professional control of crisis intervention, most other authors seem to believe that non-professional workers, or indigenous people can provide useful and quality service to the community.

The professional/non-professional controversy has implications for the definition of mental health, pathology and natural service delivery. Indigenous, naturally occurring services would not appear in incidence rates because they are responded to by the very community in which they exist without being labeled, separated, or sent off to be treated by the mental health establishment.

The definition of a person in crisis, therefore, results in part from the failure of a natural support system to succeed in helping the client manage his crisis. The oft lamented disappearance of the extended family can be seen as producing a progressive loss of a major naturally available response to people in crisis. Surprisingly television now serves as a community response to community crisis; we must think of new vehicles for crisis intervention to replace the loses produced by social change. As architects are becoming cognizant of the influence of building form on the behavior of total institution inmates, social service personnel should subject their intervention strategies to a similar kind of analysis. We are aware that today's welfare system is degrading, inefficient and anti-human, yet these services developed in response to the recognition of crises - the crises of being without food, clothing or shelter. Despite our good intentions and welfare bureaucracies, these crises persist. A memorable, scarring event in the Weisman film *Hospital* occurred when a professional mental health worker tried to assemble helpful responses to a man in crisis from the welfare bureaucracy. The frustration engendered by the immobility of the welfare agency was nearly sufficient to produce a personal crisis for the mental health worker.

If crisis intervention is viewed as an attempt to organize the immediate responsiveness of man to his distressed fellow man, then organizational structures are necessary to make that delivery more effective, predictable and of a certain quality level. It is inevitable, however, that an organization will develop structural features which serve to perpetuate the organiza-

tion and result in distortion of original service delivery goals.
Even Hotline services put together by indigenous community
people have developed elaborate structures. Over time, less
attention and manpower are devoted to the delivery of the original service and more is concentrated on determining power and
succession within the organization.

Workers interested in organizational changes and social
engineering might concentrate efforts on making complex crisis
intervention systems responsive and personal. Though large
amounts of professional manpower in helping agencies are devoted
to internal organization, staffing, funding, and budget considerations, we find that the client in crisis often faces a bewildering series of telephone operators, appointment delays,
requests for restatement of his presenting problem, and demands
for large amounts of irrelevant information. Most mental health
services are not made easily or naturally available to anyone
(this problem is not limited to the poor). Emergency crisis
centers and hotlines may have developed in direct response to
the monstrous obstacles impeding traditional mental health
delivery. It is ironic and unfortunate that, as exemplified in
the Stern chapter, such revolutionary services themselves are
beginning to develop signs of decay in the unique ability to
provide *immediate* help.

In addition to the problem of delay in service delivery,
there is the question of appropriateness. Stern acknowledges
that his crisis service is underutilized by blacks; it is evident from a careful reading of the other chapters that most of
the services described in this volume are for the middle class.
The matching of service delivery to the recipient is a concept
implied but not fully developed in the chapter by Levy. Natural-
ness, in one sense, refers to the client viewing the service as
a naturally occurring, appropriate community response to his difficulty. The arguments presented to justify the use of indigenous non-professionals have pivoted on an essential point: service provided by indigenous workers is more likely to be usable
by the client.

Unfortunately too many programs for training indigenous
workers attempt to provide trainees with skills of the trainer
and not those uniquely available to the indigenous worker. These
nonprofessionals may forsake some of the very skills which made
them initially valuable in natural service delivery. Whether
the target group is an identified minority, a racial, ethnic, or
age group, or a community, the nature of service delivery must
be consonant with that group and its values. To be effective,
crisis intervention strategies should carefully fit the ecology
of the target community. This kind of matching and exploitation

of naturally occurring resources can not usually be accomplished by an external consultant in isolation. Careful work with indigenous people is a prerequisite to effective program development. An alternative strategy is to encourage, support, and stimulate experimentation and development of totally indigenous crisis services outside the mental health framework, as exemplified by Number 9. The professional crisis intervener is not likely to be successful if he seeks to impose his view of an effective strategy for crisis intervention. Berman illustrates one way of imparting a professional perspective on crisis management without imposing rules, procedures, or technique. By helping the crisis worker experience, personally and idiosyncratically, the feeling and meaning of crisis, his responses to the person in crisis are more likely to be covariant with the emotions of the person in crisis. This matching, according to Berman, helps in crisis management.

Where is crisis intervention heading? It seems likely that there will be increasing attention to the development of immediate crisis services which can be shown to be effective in reducing the need for hospitalization. (Consider the consequences of the legislative decision in California to close most mental hospitals.) People who come up with convincing data and who appeal to the Zeitgeist will reap the necessary harvest of money and bureaucratic support. Professionals will remain the most vocal and the largest group of service providers, though indigenous and spontaneous self servicing or natural service agencies will have success in some communities. Professionals will continue to train and involve local people in first line crisis intervention.

Planning for crisis management will concentrate on "social engineering" - the design of environments to facilitate self sufficiency and interdependency. Behaviorally speaking, this will mean effective control of environments to provide reinforcers to shape and maintain competent behavior, and appropriate discriminative stimuli to signal the release of these coping behaviors. In this way, more and more naturally occurring crises (Shneidman's inter and intratemporal crises) will be reduced or met with naturally occurring community responses provided by neighbors, schools, clergy, police, social clubs, employers, and the media. Individuals in serious crisis who have not been helped sufficiently by the naturally occurring services will be directed to crisis workers.

It seems likely that the crisis mitigating resources will dramatically increase in number, variety and in unique response to community needs. As the larger communities become more complex and less responsive, spontaneous efforts to meet personal

and social crises will appear. It is not clear whether big
government will find it possible to fund many of these heretical,
unorthodox services. Government efforts are more likely to be
concentrated on the mental health establishment and on standards
of professional practice. Management by objective and cost
accounting may provide a radical challenge to traditional mental
health service delivery, but it is unlikely to provide constructive support for effective crisis intervention.

Readers of this volume are likely to have a significant
impact on the practice of crisis intervention in the decades to
come and hopefully will profit from both a close examination
and conceptual analysis of the ideas put forth herein. An understanding of the ethical and value issues implicit in service
delivery models is essential for the generation of an effective
set of crisis intervention strategies. Good research will help
answer questions about form and effect, but will not contribute
answers to ethical and value dilemmas posed by attempts at social
engineering nor resolve the conflict over the implicit models of
man represented in the differing strategies of crisis intervention. Vigilance to the consequences of crisis intervention
programs is imperative.